Integrating Complementary and Conventional Medicine

Myra Coyle-Demetriou
SRN SCM H Ed Cert Counselling Certs
Reiki Master and Holistic Therapist

and

Andrew Demetriou
MB ChB DRCOG DCH MRCGP MFHom
General Practitioner
Homeopathic Physician
Specialist Register, Faculty of Homeopathy

Foreword by
Michael Dixon
Chair, NHS Alliance

Radcliffe Publishing
Oxford • New York

Radcliffe Publishing Ltd
18 Marcham Road
Abingdon
Oxon OX14 1AA
United Kingdom

www.radcliffe-oxford.com
Electronic catalogue and worldwide online ordering facility.

British Library Cataloguing in Publication Data

A catalogue record for this book is available from the British Library.

ISBN-13: 978 184619 111 4

Typeset by Advance Typesetting Ltd, Oxford
Printed and bound by TJI Digital Ltd, Padstow, Cornwall

Conventional medicine saves life,
Complementary medicine adds quality to life.

Myra Coyle-Demetriou

As an integrated Greek doctor, it is my duty to remind you that Hippocrates is regarded as the father of modern medicine. Also, it was Hippocrates who first proposed treating 'like with like' leading to the original idea of homeopathy. So, is he also the *father* of integrated health?

Dr Andrew Demetriou
Inaugural Conference
The Prince's Foundation for Integrated Health
St James's Palace, London, 2005

Contents

Foreword   vi
About the authors   vii
Acknowledgements   viii

1   Why integrated health care?   1

PSYCHOLOGICAL ILLNESS   5
2   Anxiety   7
3   Stress   15
4   Depression   21
5   The process of death and dying   28
6   Bereavement   36

THERAPIES, HEALTH AND LIFESTYLE   43
7   Acupuncture   45
8   Aromatherapy   49
9   Ayurvedic medicine   53
10   Counselling   56
11   Herbal medicine   61
12   Homeopathy   68
13   Hypnotherapy   78
14   Massage   83
15   Meditation   87
16   Osteopathy and chiropractic: physical manipulation therapies   91
17   Prayer   97
18   Reflexology   100
19   Reiki   104
20   Traditional Chinese medicine   108
21   Yoga   111
22   Health and lifestyle   115

PHYSICAL DISEASE   123
23   Chronic disease   125
24   Dermatology   139
25   Ear, nose and throat   146
26   Headaches   155
27   Obstetrics and gynaecology   158
28   Paediatric medicine   167
29   Palliative care   174

EVALUATION AND EVIDENCE-BASED MEDICINE   179
30   Setting up an integrated health service   181
31   Evaluation   184
32   The evidence for complementary therapies   187

33   An investigation into the impact of integrating complementary
     and alternative medicine into conventional general practice   194

Index   201

Foreword

It is a real pleasure to write the foreword for this very special book. On one level it is a compendium of integrated care that covers every aspect of integration from different treatments and different diseases to research, evidence and how to provide an integrated service. On another and more practical level it will be of immense use to any clinician or patient who wishes to start on the journey towards an integrated health approach, and to those already familiar with the subject who wish to improve their skills.

In May 2006, in a speech to the World Health Organization, HRH The Prince of Wales said that integrated health care was no longer a question of 'if' but 'how' and 'how much'. With over 50% of UK general practitioners (GPs) offering patients access to complementary medicine (two-thirds in Scotland) and 75% of patients wanting complementary medicine available within the NHS, it appears that the era of integrated health care has finally arrived. Now we need to define exactly what it offers to whom and in what circumstances. That is the theme of this pioneering book. It is a map of where medicine and caring will go next, and provides a voice of hope in the future.

This is also an immensely practical book written by authors, who are themselves a conventional GP and a therapist, providing integrated care in a deprived area of Greater Manchester. For GPs and other frontline clinicians and for patients alike, it describes, for each presenting problem, the range of choices that are available for clinicians and patients pursuing an integrated approach. It opens doors and possibilities for healing that simply do not exist within a strictly conventional medical approach. I defy anyone to read the book or even just dip into it without coming away with some new tips and thoughts on healing.

Furthermore this is an extremely readable piece of work with delightful quotes and full of imaginative ideas and useful contacts within each disease area. Defying the cold rigour of a conventional textbook, it is more practical and individually useful because it embodies the warmth and experience of its authors. Integrated care is about opening the range of healing possibilities for both clinicians and patients. Individual preferences and experiences mean that response to treatment and success are bound to vary, and this represents a necessary part of the emancipating role of integrated care. So, too, is the encouragement and liberation of patients to heal themselves and also take a more active part in their own health and healing. Once a clinician or patient has embarked on this voyage, I have never known any to turn back.

The authors should be congratulated on producing such a lively and useful piece of work, which will be of practical use to every clinician and patient, whether they are experienced or are just embarking for the first time on an integrated approach to health and care.

Dr Michael Dixon
Chair, NHS Alliance
Visiting Professor, Institute of Integrated Health, Westminster University
Honorary Senior Lecturer, Peninsula Medical School
January 2007

About the authors

Myra has been married to Andrew for 30 years and they have three grown up children. She has worked in health care for most of that time, initially as a ward sister running a vascular unit and she also qualified as a midwife. Following the birth of her children, she worked in primary care with Andrew on screening programmes for the elderly, coronary heart disease (CHD) prevention and health promotion, which included stress management, exercise, health education, meditation and relaxation. She studied homeopathy, health education and counselling subsequently. For the next 14 years she worked as a counsellor in primary care in a deprived area, with special interests in health and lifestyle, bereavement, stress and anxiety management. This was followed with a keen interest in energy healing and she subsequently qualified as a Reiki master. She runs a bereavement support and marriage preparation group for her local Catholic church and continues to work as a holistic therapist to raise funds for an orphanage in Africa.

Andrew is a 1974 Liverpool Medical School graduate. As a GP principal since 1980 and a Homeopathic Physician since 1988, he gained recognition to the Specialist Register of the Faculty of Homeopathy. His main interests have been undergraduate and postgraduate teaching as a GP trainer, research and medical writing, contributing to several books and journals. He held the post of GP tutor in Bury Postgraduate Centre and with Myra runs regional workshops in the north west on motivation and prevention. He presented his research on 'Integration of Complementary Therapies in a GP Setting' at the inaugural conference of the Prince's Foundation for Integrated Health at St James's Palace. He has always emphasised the prevention and holistic aspects in his teachings and clinical care of his patients.

Acknowledgements

Our gratitude and thanks must first go to all the team at Huntley Mount Medical Centre. Their support and kindness to all, goes beyond the call of duty. They faced the task of deciphering our manuscript scribbles and tapes with great enthusiasm and endless patience. Both eyesight and computer skills were sorely tested. Thank you to Janet Morley, Maureen Foster, Denise Ives, Hilary Cornwell and also to Kath Adamson, Valerie Winstanley and June Sturman for supporting them in their task. Our appreciation must go the Association of Complementary Therapists, under the leadership of Barbara Heron, who for three years ran the scheme at our centre and helped to provide the evidence for our research study. For expert statistical analysis in Chapter 33 we are indebted to Timothy Sendall. Many thanks to Christopher Demetriou, Very Rev Paul Cannon and Sharon Beech for their expertise in computing, and for printing the many versions of the manuscript. Our gratitude and thanks to Drs Kim and Patrick Scott for their enthusiastic and painstaking reading of the book from a medical perspective.

A belated thanks goes to Andrew's grandfather, Andreas Pattichis Maos (1893–1985), who was the first to spark our interest in holistic therapy. He was a self-taught hypnotherapist of some repute, in Cyprus. A special acknowledgement must go to our children, Christopher, Lydia and Natasha, who inadvertently were guinea pigs in all our integrated and holistic ventures. A special mention to Lydia for keeping us both focused, not being afraid to speak her mind, and for setting the standard on the evidence for integrated health care. A huge debt of gratitude must go to our patients over the last 30 years for enthusiastically joining us in our quest to find appropriate integrated health care to suit their needs. We truly believe that everyone we meet is our teacher, therefore, it is a privilege to have been given the opportunity to help in some way with the health and healing process of the human condition. Our thanks to Gillian Nineham, Jamie Etherington and Radcliffe Publishing Ltd for having the vision and respect for the subject matter and for publishing *Integrating Complementary and Conventional Medicine*.

To both sets of parents, who have now passed on, we dedicate this book for their part in our journey. For our children, Christopher, Lydia and Natasha, who are blessed with a beautiful spirit. To our 24 children that we 'adopted' in Africa, who struggle daily for their survival and an uncertain future.

Why integrated health care?

Have a mind that is open to everything and attached to nothing.

Wayne Dyer[1]

Integration is the holistic approach to health care using conventional and complementary therapies, bringing the human touch back to modern medicine.

This book is written from the perspective that a medical diagnosis is already established. It is envisaged that the information is used to consider appropriate integration using various therapies and treatments: a combination that provides a truly integrated healthcare system – the marriage of complementary and conventional medicine.

By optimising effectiveness and minimising side-effects, we demonstrate how this can also be cost-effective. The information obtained from this holistic approach, we hope, will inspire further reading, creating awareness and interest in the therapeutic processes from the different disciplines and medical approaches from around the world. It can also be used as a practical guide for referral, recommending or dealing with a patient's enquiry as to whether a particular therapy is appropriate.

It is our hope and expectation that other health professionals will be interested enough to find the guidance they need to set up an integrated health care service.

Each section has been set out in a format that will make the information practical and easy to assimilate.

This is an overview and a practical guide to integrated medicine; 'a picture of holism'.

The *'art' of integration* is demonstrated throughout the book. We hope that *our* enthusiasm becomes *your* enthusiasm.

The aims of this book

The aims of the book are to:

- teach new skills
- encourage professional training in complementary medicine
- refer patients to complementary practitioners
- understand the potential benefits of these therapies
- raise awareness of the use of therapies by patients
- integrate therapies into existing health services for wider patient choice
- demonstrate a holistic approach to prevention and disease management
- show the potential for reducing general practitioner (GP) workload (*see* Chapter 31)
- create an awareness of the potential healing power in every human being.

For the patient, who may want to seek complementary input as part of their long-term care plan following a medical diagnosis, this information will help them to decide which therapy is appropriate. Some of the commonest conditions are discussed in each section, providing the opportunity for self-help. Most patients prefer to be actively involved in their care and are also keen for a proactive approach to aid their recovery.

Integrated medicine adds quality to health care, enhances the healing process, provides more choice and gives responsibility back to the patient.

> *The Life so short, the craft so long to learn.*
>
> *Hippocrates*

Building a bridge between complementary and conventional medicine

Many areas in modern medicine can incorporate complementary principles in order to stimulate the body's own healing abilities and enhance the quality of care. One such example is to use complementary therapies in self-limiting illness to reduce antibiotic prescribing in order to minimise drug resistance.

The 'one size fits all' teaching of conventional medicine is not always appropriate, whereas complementary medicine embraces the diversity of the individuals' make-up and recognises that different techniques and treatments are needed for individual personality types. This is no better illustrated than in homeopathy.

Limitations in conventional research need to be recognised and taken into account in the design of studies involving complementary therapies, and more research funding made available.

- Surveys have shown that 75% of the population in the UK want complementary therapies to be available on the NHS, and that 20 million people, one-third of the population, have used complementary medicine (*see* Chapter 32).
- Research has shown that 50% of general practices offer or refer to complementary therapists (*see* Chapter 32).
- Practice-based commissioning (PBC) is a realistic option for funding.
- In the UK, 50 universities are now teaching complementary medicine.

> *Complacency is the enemy of study. We cannot really learn anything until we rid ourselves of complacency. Our attitude towards ourselves should be 'to be insatiable in learning', and towards others 'to be tireless in teaching'.*
>
> *Chairman Mao*[2]

The holistic approach should be the foundation of every healthcare intervention, restoring the human factor to modern medicine. Doctors are well placed to facilitate and harness the healing process.

> *Change is but an attitudinal step away.*
>
> *David Brooks*[3]

How to use this book

The book has been divided into four sections:

- Psychological illness
- Therapies, health and lifestyle
- Physical disease
- Evaluation and evidence-based medicine.

Psychological illness and physical disease

Each medical condition demonstrates the place of complementary therapies in the treatment process within integrated health care. Therapies that are most commonly used are described in the context of the disease process.

Therapies

This section provides a synopsis of the mainstream complementary therapies and describes the essential elements of each. Details for contacting organisations involved in training can also be found, to enable the reader to gain further information. This section will give an insight into understanding the historical background, application and the evidence for the effectiveness of each treatment or therapy.

Evaluation and evidence-based medicine

Throughout all the sections, references and further reading are included to enable more detailed study of each discipline. The importance of evaluation and evidence-based medicine is also emphasised. In the final chapter a three-year outcome study is included not only as an illustration of effectiveness but also an example of integration of complementary therapies into a National Health Service (NHS) practice. The research study is entitled 'An investigation into the impact of integrating complementary and alternative medicine into conventional general practice' (*see* Chapter 33).

This book is intended for doctors, nurses, therapists, and patients.

Our spheres of experience reflect our own professional interest in Reiki energy healing, counselling, nursing, midwifery, general practice and homeopathy. We therefore make no apology for emphasising these areas in our presentation of integrated health care.

The names of patients in case studies throughout the book have been changed for confidentiality.

References

1   Dyer W. *10 Secrets for Success and Inner Peace*. London: Hay House; 2005.
2   Piao L. *Quotations from Chairman Mao Tse-Tung*. 2nd edn. Peking: Foreign Languages Press; 1967.
3   Brooks D. Teams for tomorrow towards a new primary care system. *J RCGP* 1986; 36: 285–6.

Psychological illness

Anxiety

The demand for a false self to cover and hide the authentic self necessities a life dominated by doing and achievement.

John Bradshaw[1]

Anxiety

This is a modern day 'plague', which robs us of our peace of mind and is often used to describe a specific set of symptoms. No two people display exactly the same physical or emotional problems; we all react very differently depending on our individual make-up. Most anxious people describe a distressing feeling of uneasiness or dread. The fear may be rational, irrational or of an anticipated event which may or may not take place.

A certain amount of unrealistic and irrational anxiety is part of most people's experience, hence it is an expected normal functioning of the human personality. It is termed as chronic when the anxiety is not traceable to any specific cause or trigger and interferes with normal functional daily activity. Anxious people are in a state of suspense, always waiting 'for something to happen', with a watchful awareness and alertness, over-sensitivity to noise and often helplessness in the face of perceived danger. There is fear of the future, the 'what if' or 'just in case', the need to try to anticipate the fear in advance in order to feel better, as in perfectionist behaviour. In the long term with this scenario, all energy is spent on the prevention of fear to satisfy the 'just in case', like a cat chasing its tail. Anxiety can be felt acutely in the morning following sleep, or in early morning waking. The physical symptoms are many and varied, for example headaches, backache, irritable bowel syndrome, insomnia, lack of concentration and so forth. Often, these symptoms are treated individually without a holistic approach to determine the root cause. Fear and love are the main heartfelt emotions that seem to dominate our lives.

Counselling highlights awareness of personal power and effective control, but equally helps deal with unresolved issues that caused the anxiety. It can also enable a change of attitudes and negativity and replace these with a more positive approach. Ultimately, the patient can achieve a sense of balance and acquire strategies to use for their long-term health and 'wellbeing' (*see* Chapter 10). Fear can often manifest in obsessions and phobias. Anxiety and mental health issues form around 40% of the workload in primary care.[2] Management is usually by drug therapy in the first instance. It can make patients dependent on medication and the doctor. This often leaves both the doctor and patient feeling frustrated at the lack of sustainable progress.

Integrated management of this fear seeks to educate the patient about their anxiety and how they can manage their own fears and worries. In doing so, this puts the power where it should be, with the patient, who can then take personal responsibility for their feelings and general 'wellbeing'. We do not have a choice about what happens in our life, but we do have a choice in how we deal with it.

Management

The integrated approach to long-term care is based on:

- *awareness*: of the condition and its effects
- *reassurance*: by excluding any physical cause
- *dealing with symptoms*: such as headaches and sweating
- *long-term plan*: for example relaxation classes, yoga, meditation, lifestyle change and self-help.

Proactive and symptomatic control approach
Physical exercise (*see* Chapter 22)

Physical activity will help to deal with some of the symptoms of anxiety and balance energy levels from mental activity to the physical body. It will also rid the system of the end-products of the adrenaline build-up.

Counselling and psychotherapy (*see* Chapter 10)

This is helpful when there are psychological problems, as a result of physical, emotional and sexual abuse. Patients with a history of rape or anorexia nervosa may also benefit from group work as part of their long-term care plan.

Homeopathy

Homeopathy in the management of anxiety is without risk of addiction and has no side-effects. Some of the remedies that can help in anxiety are as follows:

- *Avena sativa*: aids sleep and helps with relaxation
- *Arsenicum*: reduces fear, prevents panic
- *Lycopodium*: deals with apprehension
- *Argentum nitricum*: for exam fears/stage fright
- *Staphysagria*: for anger management
- *Aconite napellis and Ignatia*: to reduce the effects of panic attacks
- *Gelsemium*: helps with intense fear for no apparent reason.

Diet (*see* Chapter 22)

- *Eating regularly* is essential to avoid hypoglycaemic attacks and to help concentration. A three-hourly balanced diet is therefore beneficial.
- *Avoiding tea, coffee and alcohol*: these are stimulants and can have an adverse effect on an already stressed system. Replacing these with herbal teas and fresh juices and increasing water intake (2 litres of fluid daily) helps the recovery process.

- *Supplements*: in chronic anxiety, because of the constant tension held in the body, depletion can take place of calcium, zinc and vitamin C; evening primrose oil and omega 3 are also useful supplements.

Lifestyle management (*see* Chapter 22)

To achieve a balance for maintaining 'wellbeing', it is beneficial to use the basic, **24-hour cycle of life indicator: 8 hours' good work, 8 hours' relaxation and 8 hours' sleep.**
  If we live by this simple principle it will enable us to keep healthy in mind, body and spirit and to become more effective individuals.

> *We must remember all our lives to raise our heads and be aware of the horizon.*
> *Frank Delaney*[3]

Reiki

Reiki is a form of hands-on energy healing and is invaluable in balancing the negative energy created by high levels of anxiety. Peace of mind is often difficult to achieve even for a short time. This healing energy calms the tension, creating a feeling of relaxation that helps to induce sleep, which can be difficult to achieve even with hypnotics. The recommended schedule is one-hour sessions on a weekly basis for at least 4 weeks. Anxious people quite often forget what it feels like to be relaxed, and Reiki reminds them of the calmness that can be achieved (*see* Chapter 19).

Case study 2.1

Mary is a 43-year-old lady, who lives with her teenage son and elderly mother. She was assaulted in a car park, sustaining multiple soft tissue injuries including a fracture of her cricoid bone, sprained left wrist and left ankle. She had difficulty in mobilising, needing crutches initially. Mary's disturbed sleep became problematic; she also suffered with panic attacks and was frightened of leaving the house. She was given Ruta and Arnica homeopathic remedies for bruising and pain relief to take for four weeks. Mary received counselling and Reiki healing, which helped to calm her anxieties and induced sleep. She had six one-hourly sessions on a weekly basis. She then returned to work soon afterwards and was promoted to a new position at the top of her profession.

Case study 2.2

John is a 61 year old who presented with a lifelong anxiety, suffered stress at work and could no longer cope. His father was very strict with him, and he said that as a boy 'nothing he did was ever good enough'. He admitted to being a 'perfectionist' and difficult to live with. He developed a transient ischaemic attack and had great difficulty sleeping. He also had high blood pressure. John lost all his confidence and was so anxious he stopped driving. He managed within 2 months to control his anxiety through stress counselling and the help of six sessions of Reiki healing. He returned to work able to drive and coping well again. His blood pressure settled to within normal range. On review one year later his improvement was maintained.

Panic attacks

A panic attack is a severe bout of anxiety, fear that occurs quite often without warning and with no apparent trigger factor. Around one in ten people suffer from these extremely frightening and debilitating attacks.[4] It is a physical manifestation of what is happening in the mind. When the body reacts like this it tends to develop a pattern or an imprint and becomes conditioned to reacting in a particular way. This behaviour often occurs when it is least expected, when the mind is in a relaxed state and it does not 'feel' logical to the person who is suffering, therefore the fear is all the greater. Negative energy, when not being channelled out of the body into work or exercise, has a huge effect on the system because of the adrenaline surge, and can cause a virtual 'paralysis'. Panic attacks can have quite extreme symptoms, from the usual dizziness, nausea, sweating, fainting and palpitations to rapid breathing, tachycardia, chest pain, muscle cramps and exhaustion. Irrational fear takes many forms, and phobias are a fairly common presentation. This can be triggered by objects or situations such as spiders, flying, heights, being in crowded or closed up spaces (claustrophobia) or finding it hard to leave the house (agoraphobia).

Management

Investigations

Investigations are necessary to rule out any pathology if there is any doubt about the diagnosis. A full blood count and thyroid function tests should be included and, if indicated, an electrocardiogram (ECG) recording. This will often help to reassure the patient.

Breathing techniques

Breathing techniques can provide immediate care to help control attacks. Patients can easily be taught this simple technique. Breathing is an automatic survival mechanism. We cannot live without drawing breath, but there is a right and efficient way, and a wrong and inefficient way. During stressful times we tend to **overbreathe.** This is part of the stress response, but unfortunately it can increase our distress. When we breathe rapidly from our upper chest, because there is no physical outlet hyperventilation occurs, which means there is an imbalance between carbon dioxide and oxygen, increasing the fear, resulting in a rapid pulse, muscle cramps, pins and needles and numbness. Anxious people tend to breathe rapidly and talk as they breathe. This long-term inefficient breathing can create chronic emotional and physical health problems. **It is important to inform the patient that normal breathing consists of a stationary chest, and an abdomen that** moves outward when breathing in and inwards when breathing out. To practise doing this, the right hand is placed on the chest and the left hand on the abdomen. This simple technique is useful in **panic attacks** and **hyperventilation** to calm and relax the mind and body. The focus is always brought back to the breathing, the technique can be used on a daily basis before, during and after stressful events and situations.

Counselling and anxiety management

This is essential to prevent attacks occurring in the future (*see* Chapter 10).

Behavioural therapy

This can help the patient learn how to change behaviour and to 'feel the fear and do it anyway', which can, with enough personal emotional experiences, lead to desensitisation.

Homeopathic treatment

Examples of remedies that can help are:

- *Passiflora*: for a calming effect
- *Avena sativa*: this helps to aid sleep
- *Ignatia*: for changing emotions
- *Aconite napellis*: for fear and panic
- *Lycopodium*: for anticipation and in early morning waking.

Relaxation measures

Examples of therapies that help are Reiki healing (*see* Chapter 19), meditation (Chapter 15), yoga (Chapter 21) and hypnotherapy (*see* Chapter 13).

Diet

- This is discussed earlier in this chapter in 'Anxiety' (*see* p. 8), and in Chapter 22.

Avoidance of stress overload

An awareness of our own personal emotional limitations will often prevent a crisis. Taking stock of life events and their cumulative effects and learning to reduce potential stressors can prevent health problems arising.

Obsessive–compulsive behaviour

Obsessions are thoughts or ideas that persistently seize the mind and will not let go. The compulsive part of the syndrome is the irresistible urge to act on a thought or idea. The type of person who displays this behaviour feels driven to perform or act on these thoughts, which are usually persistent, difficult to control and unwelcome.

The two disorders of obsession and compulsion are often associated and are known as an obsessive–compulsive disorder. For example, hypochondria is an obsession with health. Individuals with this condition usually have a stock of medicines at home, rather like a mini-pharmacy, and are always following the latest health trends. To some degree, this behaviour is accepted as normal in the human population at large. Anorexia is an obsession with physical appearance but is often gauged by the sufferer as a controlling mechanism. It is about satisfying the compulsion, as a need for peace of mind. It tends to focus on starving the body to achieve perfection, in order to feel good. Low self-esteem and depression are major factors in this condition. Most people have some simple and harmless obsessions and compulsions, mainly to do with diet, health, personal safety, or in keeping fit. It becomes a problem only when the behaviour dominates and disrupts normal life, and severe mental health problems can ensue. In most cases, obsessive–compulsive behaviour is a result of anxiety, and may be rooted in the subconscious, which may be based in fear that something bad will happen if the action of the thought or idea is not carried out. As an example, a person may feel compelled to wash their hands, body or clothes in case they contract an infection or disease. If, for whatever reason, this act cannot be carried out, then the anxiety levels rise and they become overwhelmed with fear. It is then a battleground for control and becomes obsessive and compulsive. The sufferer is driven to keep control of their place in the world at any cost. This of course is only a short-term means of handling the anxiety by acting on the thought process. The Beck Anxiety Inventory has been found to be useful in screening and measurement of this aspect of anxiety.[5]

Management

Management sometimes requires specialist skills depending on the degree of the illness.

Referral to a psychiatrist/psychologist

It is often necessary to refer to a specialist with an interest in this area of emotional dysfunction.

Behavioural therapy

This can help to educate the sufferer to manage the anxiety longer-term and hopefully learn that 'nothing bad will happen and that the irrational fears do not come true'. The cycle of fear needs to be broken.

Homeopathy

These are some examples of common remedies used:[6]

- *Avena sativa*: this tincture helps with relaxation and induces sleep
- *Aurum met*: this is useful when there are thoughts of death and dying
- *Thuja*: this is used when there is a compulsion to touch things
- *Silica*: used when the patient counts things obsessively
- *Arsenicum*: this is mostly used when there is a degree of perfectionism.

Relaxation classes (see Chapter 22)

Participation in activities such as yoga (*see* Chapter 21), meditation (*see* Chapter 15) or Reiki healing sessions (*see* Chapter 19) can be of benefit to help achieve a relaxed state, to balance the fear and take control.

Physical exercise (see Chapter 22)

Physical activity directs the emotional energy of fear into physical energy, creating a balance and a more natural tiredness.

Diet

A balanced diet is essential in order to control the anxiety by maintaining blood sugar levels, helping to promote sleep, and is also useful in the control of panic attacks (*see* Chapter 22).

> *Quiet minds cannot be perplexed or frightened, but go on in fortune or misfortune at their own private pace, like a clock in a thunderstorm.*
>
> *Robert Louis Stevenson*[7]

References

1 Bradshaw J. *Healing the Shame that Binds You* Deerfield Beach, FL: Health Communications, Inc; 1988.
2 Ronalds C, Kapur N, Stone K *et al*. Determinants of consultation rate in patients with anxiety and depressive disorders in primary care. *Fam Pract* 2002; 19: 23–8.
3 Delaney F. *A Novel Ireland*. London: Time Warner Books; 2004.
4 Birchall H, Brandon S and Taub N. Panic in a general practice population: prevalence, psychiatric co-morbidity and associated disability. *Soc Psychiatry Psychiatr Epidemiol* 2000; 35: 235–41.
5 Leyfer OT, Ruberg JL and Woodruff-Borden J. Examination of the utility of the Beck Anxiety Inventory and its factors as a screener for anxiety disorders. *J Anxiet Disord* 2006; 20: 444–58.
6 McCutcheon LE. Treatment of anxiety with a homeopathic remedy. *J Appl Nutr* 1996; 48: 2–6.
7 Stevenson RL. *An Inland Voyage*. Whitefish, MT: Kessinger Publishing; 2004.

Further reading

- Bloom W. *The Endorphin Effect: a breakthrough strategy for holistic health and spiritual wellbeing*. London: Piatkus; 2000.
- Holford P. *The Optimum Nutrition Bible*. London: Piatkus; 1997.
- McGraw C. *Self Matters, Creating Your Life from the Inside Out*. London: Simon and Schuster; 2002.
- Payne R. *Relaxation Techniques*. London: Churchill Livingstone; 1995.
- Pert CB. *Molecules of Emotion: why you feel the way you feel*. New York: Simon and Schuster; 1997.
- Subby R. *Healing the Family Within*. Florida: Health Communications Inc; 1990.
- Walker M. *Women in Therapy and Counselling*. Milton Keynes: Open University Press; 1990.

Contacts

- *Mind (mental health charity)*: www.mind.org.uk; tel: 020 8519 2122
- *Relationship counselling (Relate)*: www.relate.org.uk
- *Triumph Over Phobia*: www.triumphoverphobia.com; tel: 01225 330353
- *United Kingdom Council for Psychotherapists*: www.psychotherapy.org.uk; tel: 020 7436 3002

3

Stress

Men are disturbed not by things, but by the views which they take of them.

Epictetus

Stress is a normal healthy part of everyday life. It is the result of interactive behaviour between people and their environment and it is a unique experience for the individual. A situation that is stressful for one person can be a positive experience for another. It is a basic human instinct and reaction, a defence mechanism against harm and a survival tool. The stress response prepares the body for physical activity. **It is defined as a state we experience when there is a disparity between how we view demands and how we think we can cope with their expectations.**

Stress can also be the result of sudden change, which we can never really be prepared for; often 'blind panic' can follow as a result, as part of the **fight or flight response**. Our ancestors used this reaction to survive in the wild; it was essential for human survival, a choice to stand and physically fight or have the speed and strength to run away. Signals from the brain indicate a need to respond. This message is then relayed to the suprarenals, where noradrenaline, adrenaline and cortisol are released to deal with the perceived threat. This is necessary in order for an appropriate reaction to take place for human survival.

We of course are not in the same league as that of our ancestors in terms of need, but we are bombarded psychologically from many different angles in today's society. Fearfulness can arise from financial insecurity, emotional instability, lack of self-esteem, or in questioning our place in society. Relationships with partners, family and friends, not to mention surviving in the workplace, all require balancing. We have so many different and difficult areas of daily existence to contend with. Modern society has high expectations of the human condition. Everyone is chasing after the perceived good life, individuals do expect more today and competition is greater. Our stress response is being constantly activated. We so easily become addicted to a high state of stress alert, and unfortunately there are not enough outlets for the frustration, anger, disappointments and injustices that ensue. We need to proactively work on a regular de-stressing regime that is suited to our particular needs and personality. Quite often, finding the ability to put the emotion of the situation on the 'back burner' and the practical use of logic can defuse many stressful situations.

It is requisite for relaxation of the mind that we make use, from time to time, of playful deeds and jokes.

Thomas Aquinas (1225–1274)

Around three-quarters of all medical consultations in primary care also have a stress-related component, such as alcohol and drug abuse, migraine, tension headaches, irritable bowel syndrome, dyspepsia, hypertension, anxiety, depression and phobias, to name but a few.[1] Many reactions to everyday stresses will depend on learnt behaviour from parents, peer groups and from social background 'norms'. How consistently difficult situations were handled, and the individual's own abilities in dealing with these are significant factors in dealing with stress.

This recognised modern phenomenon of stress is a very popular concept, and most people are comfortable in relating to this and are happy to talk about the condition. Stress is not associated with the taboo of depression, and it is perceived as a busy and popular person's condition until it affects an individual's health.

Managing stress is ultimately a personal responsibility. The emphasis is on helping patients to recognise the stressor, given their ability, and helping them to deal with it in an impartial and appropriate way. Nature has its own way of recharging our energy levels. We need to learn to harness nature's bounty on a regular basis and in terms of need. Every action, conscious or unconscious, has the ability to use stored energy, which comes from our natural ability for body repair. Real relaxation is truly experienced by mind and body when little or no energy has been expended. Even simple things like decision making in daily life as well as in the workplace can cause stress, because of the potential conflict element and the way that difficult events are perceived and interpreted. On the positive side, the 'feel good factor' of a communication well done, having 'said what needed to be said, listened and been listened to', with self-esteem intact, is a very positive result and a great confidence booster, balancing the positive and the negative.

Stress is linked to lowered immunity, including increased susceptibility to infection, a greater propensity for relapse of chronic inflammatory conditions, a poor response to immunisations and altered patterns of allergic reaction to stress, and also to distressing memory impairment.[2] This very much depends on the individual's emotional reaction to stress and the extent to which there is a feeling of personal control of the situation in hand.

Stress symptoms

- Lethargy and tiredness
- Insomnia
- Restlessness
- Headaches
- Irritable bowel syndrome, diarrhoea or constipation
- Tearfulness
- Inability to finish tasks
- Palpitations
- Irritability
- Fault finding
- Feeling overwhelmed, an inability to cope
- Exacerbation of existing medical problems

Life events that often cause stress

- Death of a spouse or child
- Divorce
- Marital separation

- Death of family or friend
- Personal injury or chronic ill-health
- Job loss through redundancy or being dismissed
- Retirement
- House move or moving out of an area
- New baby
- Major disaster
- Unbalanced lifestyle

Positive outcomes of stress

- Excitement
- Productivity
- Stimulation
- Creativity
- Achievement
- Confidence building
- Educating
- Harmony
- Fun

Negative results of stress

Stress affects us all in many ways, for example emotionally, psychologically and physically. Where pressure and a sense of failure predominate day-to-day living, this creates disharmony and feelings of anger, anxiety and depression. In the longer-term, this may result in physical ill-health such as duodenal ulcers, heart problems, and lowered immunity levels. Prolonged stress can lead to a nervous breakdown and possible suicide.

Stress management

Conventional medical approach

This is sometimes necessary in treating symptoms, and may include hypnotics, anxiolytics and tranquillisers.

Breathing technique

See Chapter 2 (p. 10) for explanation and method. Knowing how to control breathing is the basis for relaxation.

Developing daily routines

These make life less frenetic and more ordered and also help an individual to regain control of the situation in order to relax and achieve peace of mind. Meditation (*see* Chapter 15) practised regularly is beneficial for mind control at all times. Yoga is a complete mind and body tool suitable for everyone as a means to de-stress, and can easily be included in a daily routine (*see* Chapter 21).[3] It is also beneficial to develop hobbies that regularly take the mind away from the stressor.

Physical exercise

This is a positive means for the body to de-stress, rebalancing energy levels from the mental to the physical. Physical activity also aids sleep and reinforces the 'feel good factor', giving a sense of achievement (*see* Chapter 22).

Homeopathic remedies

These are often based on individual personalities (constitutional remedies):

- *Coffea cruda*: this remedy can be helpful for the overactive mind
- *Avena sativa*: this is useful in insomnia and for relaxation
- *Lycopodium*: for fear and apprehension and irritable bowel syndrome
- *Sulphur*: to help anxiety in a sulphur type patient
- *Nux vomica*: can help irritability and control anger
- *Arsenicum*: used in perfectionism.

Diet

A well-balanced diet full of fresh produce is essential, with added vitamin C, garlic, omega 3, calcium, magnesium and zinc for women particularly, because long-term stress may have an effect on lowering levels (*see* Chapter 22).

Lifestyle

It is important to create a balance in 24-hour cycle where there is: **8 hours' work, 8 hours' relaxation and 8 hours' sleep** (*see* Chapter 22). It is also of value to create a lifestyle that suits the personality.

Assertiveness training and attitude awareness

This highlights behaviour, for stress awareness, and helps people become more effective by teaching the importance of:

- *self-awareness*: of one's own goals, behaviour, openness, honesty, integrity and intuition
- *self-acceptance*: with positive self-regard
- *empathy and acceptance*: with an understanding of others from an individual perspective
- *gratitude*: for our many blessings.

Other helpful factors

- Developing a sense of humour
- Learning to say 'no'
- Delegating, when the going gets tough
- Organising, prioritising from most important to least important
- Working efficiently, using a diary and keeping to it
- Avoiding uncertainty and using realistic goals
- Avoiding perfectionism and being happy with your best
- Finding work that suits your personality
- Talking and sharing with friends and colleagues in the same position
- Finding emotional support in a partner, parents, friends or agency

---

Case study 3.1

John, a 40-year-old businessman who felt stressed and anxious, drank a lot of coffee to 'keep him going' and subsequently had difficulty sleeping. His wife was worried, because he was often very irritable and started losing his temper more than usual. His blood pressure was also high and he was sweating when resting. Work became very busy and he had difficulty turning down lucrative contracts. John was given Aconite napellis, a homeopathic remedy, for when he felt anxious and frightened. Nux vomica was given for the irritability, and Sulphur to reduce his blood pressure. His coffee intake was reduced to one cup a day. He attended six sessions of Reiki, which consisted of a one-hour session each week and counselling. John also took up fishing as a hobby to help him to relax. His job was physically demanding, so he needed to rest more; after a few weeks he was much improved. He continued to have Reiki healing and counselling on a monthly basis. His blood pressure returned to normal, his sleep had improved and he became much more efficient at work. The most important factors for him were being aware of his stressor, learning to manage his stress levels, and becoming more effective in his work situation.

The greater the obstacle the more glory in overcoming it.

Molière

References

1 Zamtinge EM, Verhaak PFM and Benfing JM. The workload of GPs: patients with psychological and somatic problems compared. *Fam Pract* 2005; 22: 293–7.
2 Newcomer JW, Selke G, Melson AK *et al*. Decreased memory performance in healthy humans induced by stress-level cortisol treatment. *Arch Gen Psychiatry* 1999; 56: 527–33.
3 Michalsen A, Grossman P, Acil A *et al*. Rapid stress reduction and anxiolysis among distressed women as a consequence of a three-month intensive yoga program. *Med Sci Monit* 2005; 11: 555–61.

Further reading

- Bloom W. *The Endorphin Effect; a Breakthrough Strategy for Holistic Health and Well-being*. London: Piatkus; 2000.
- Greener M. *The Which Guide to Managing Stress*. London: Which Book Consumer Association; 1996.
- Holford P. *The Optimum Nutrition Bible*. London: Piatkus; 1997.
- Muir A and Humbly N. *Stress Management in Primary Care*. London: Butterworth-Heinemann; 1997.
- Payne R. *Relaxation Techniques*. London: Churchill Livingstone; 1995.

Contacts

- *Action on Smoking and Health*: www.ash.org.uk
- *Health and Lifestyle issues*: www.bbc.co.uk/health/mental/stress.shtml
- *International Stress Management Association (UK)*: www.isma.org.uk
- *Mind (mental health charity)*: www.mind.org.uk; tel: 020 8519 2122
- *On Nutrition*: www.mynutrition.co.uk

4

Depression

Medicine seeks to heal the body without recognising the energy of the soul,
psychology seeks to heal the personality without recognising the force of the soul,
that lies behind the configuration and experience of personality and therefore,
also cannot heal at the level of the soul.

Gary Zukav[1]

Depression is a very common condition, which affects people all over the world. The European Outcome of Depression International Network (ODIN) study gave an overall prevalence of depressive disorders of 8.6%. For women the rate was 10.6% and for men 6.6%.[2] This condition can affect anyone, young or old, it has no social boundaries. The highest rates in the European study were in cities in the UK and Ireland, and the lowest rate was in urban Spain. Depression and mental health problems generally still have a stigma attached, with a very negative label and a sense of personal failure. The word depression, even in our modern 21st century, conjures up a fear of psychiatrists, asylums and conditions that in the past were very much taboo in society, and can still inject the same dread today. In comparison, the word 'stress' has a more modern feel to it. It is more acceptable to be stressed as it conjures up images of hard work and being in demand, popular and conscientious, which is much more open to discussion. It can therefore be very difficult for the sufferer to admit to the condition at one level and to establish the symptoms as being those of depression. This is because many of the signs are physical, and the investigations quite often take this path.

Depression is classified as mild, moderate and severe, with many variations in between. Some people live with a mild form of depression. They know how to deal with it, for example a change of scene, holidays, exercise, lifestyle change, talking it over with someone, positive thinking and generally finding ways to lift their mood. The depressed mind can switch into automatic behaviour so that it can become locked into a control scenario, which displays rather fixed ideas and beliefs, leading to anger, fear, guilt or into a very negative way of processing thoughts. Hopelessness and despair often set in, and in turn this affects the mind, body and spirit. When this complicated cycle of negativity is established, management and treatment are needed to help change this pattern. Drug therapy alone may not cure depression but will often reduce some of the symptoms; however as soon as the drugs are withdrawn the negativity may return if the root cause is not properly dealt with.

Depression can be divided into two main types. The first is reactive, which follows the many life changes for example the death of a loved one, ill-health (such as cancer, heart problems or stroke), divorce or separation. The condition can also arise as the result of major mental or physical trauma. The second is endogenous depression. This is the result of a biochemical imbalance, which can produce periods of euphoria or mania as well as the complete opposite of extremely low moods. It can change from sadness to complete hopelessness with a huge complexity of physical symptoms. Anxiety can quite often mask a depressed state, especially if there is a major physical or emotional trauma. Women present more often than men for treatment; however, in females this can often be masked by a hormone imbalance, for example premenstrual syndrome or menopause.

Our sense of self is often related to our feeling of being the same person for the whole of our lives, a necessary sense of continuity. Experiences, positive or negative, shape the choices we make and actions we take at any given time. Memories can be reconstructed, distorted and repressed completely. The exposure of repressed memories can, of course, help psychological and emotional recovery. A stable and intact memory indicates a sense of 'wellbeing'. Loss of memory due to aging, shock, stress, and depression is quite common. To have an understanding of the basis and need for continuity of this sense of who we are will help to shape our decision in terms of caring for individuals holistically.

Chemical and biological problems that can cause mood swings

- Anaemia
- Hypothyroidism
- Menopause
- Premenstrual syndrome
- Drugs and alcohol addiction
- Postnatal problems
- Glandular fever
- Vitamin deficiency such as vitamin B6
- Use of the combined oral contraceptive pill

These biological and chemical causes have to be investigated and treated appropriately with the help of integrated medicine.

> *Happiness resides not in possessions and not in gold,*
> *the feeling of happiness dwells in the Soul.*
>
> *Democritus*

Symptoms of depression

Symptoms of depression can include:

- feeling down/low mood
- recurrent thoughts of suicide
- self-harm
- indecision
- lack of interest
- weight loss or weight gain
- slowing down
- insomnia
- lack of energy
- tearfulness, sighing

- a feeling of being disconnected from reality
- memory loss and confusion
- negative attitude generally.

Management of depression

Shared medical management with a psychiatrist or psychologist is essential with the more severe depressive states such as manic depression, schizophrenia, suicidal patients and major degrees of postnatal depression. Alcohol-dependence syndromes and drug addiction usually involve the community alcohol drug team in the first instance. Good communication between all disciplines of care is necessary in order to promote recovery to full functional and enjoyable mental and physical health.

Counselling and psychotherapy

It is important to get to the root of the problem and unravel the past to prevent chronic ill-health (*see* Chapter 10) and learn to take responsibility for emotional 'wellbeing'.

Relaxation therapies

Examples include acupuncture (*see* Chapter 7), meditation (*see* Chapter 15), aromatherapy (*see* Chapter 8), massage (*see* Chapter 14), Reiki healing (*see* Chapter 19) and health and lifestyle (*see* Chapter 22). The above therapies are beneficial in helping to rebalance the system, regain a sense of perspective and increase energy levels.

Herbal medicine

Herbal remedies are useful, for example St John's wort (Hypericum perforatum) (*see* Chapter 11) is well known, has been proven effective and can be bought over the counter.

Diet

A regular diet with increased fresh fruit and vegetables is essential for recovery. Often there is a great disinterest in healthy foods, with a tendency to indulge in comfort eating (*see* Chapter 22).

Homeopathy

A few remedies are listed as examples that can be used on their own or with allopathic medicines (*see* Chapter 12).

- *Sepia*: for feeling tearful, irritable, chilly, everything is an effort
- *Aurum*: for feeling worthless, suicidal
- *Ignatia*: following grief
- *Natrum muriaticum*: for bottled up emotions

- *Staphysagria*: used in anger, resentment
- *Calcarea carbonica*: useful in sleep disturbances
- *Nux vomica*: for those who are extremely irritable with 'fault finding' behaviour
- *Lycopodium*: for an extremely haughty personality who is constantly worried with early morning waking

(**Note**: all the above remedies help with sleep disturbance.)

Lifestyle

Sometimes, a simple change in lifestyle, emotional support and a positive outlook is all that is needed for healing and recovery to take place (*see* Chapter 22).

Laughter therapy

The therapeutic effects of good humour improve the general outlook of the negative personality, which is essential to help control depression. It is thought to:

- relax the muscles
- aid mental and physical healing
- relieve pain
- reduce stress
- improve circulation
- improve concentration
- lower blood pressure
- balance perspectives
- calm the mind
- have no known side-effects.

> *A merry heart does good like a medicine, but a broken spirit dries the bones.*
> *Proverbs 17:22*

The ability to laugh at one's self, situations or problems makes life much easier and gives less of an emotional power to the situation, hence affording the ability to see it for what it is. Humour can increase the positive and hopeful attitudes and dispel feelings of depression and helplessness. Laughter will release the tension that otherwise would be held like a vice in the body, leading to long-term problems.

> *Our greatest discovery is that we can alter our lives by altering our attitudes. It is*
> *your thought life, not your circumstances that determines your happiness.*
> *Philippians 2:5*

Exercise (see Chapter 22)

Using exercise to improve and boost a patient's mood is proving to have huge benefits for clients with low mood.[3] Exercise is known to raise the brain's level of dopamine, serotonin and noradrenaline, all neurotransmitters that affect mood. These are the same chemicals that are controlled by antidepressant medication. Professor Ellen Billett at the sports science department of Nottingham Trent University has found that levels of phenylethylamine, which is similar in structure to amphetamine, increased substantially during a workout, to produce a significant mood-busting effect.[4]

The Mental Health Foundation of Britain is running a campaign to raise awareness of these benefits in helping to treat mild to moderate depression. Around three million people in the UK suffer from mental ill-health; it is also one of the commonest medical conditions in the UK. The British Mental Health Foundation believes 'exercise schemes give people contact and motivation, which can boost their recovery'.[4]

Case study 4.1

Jean is a 55-year-old lady who has suffered from depression since her husband died 4 years previously. She also suffered from seasonal affect disorder (SAD) for many years. Jean became very anergic and felt 'disconnected'. She would cook all her meals for the week in advance. This was in case she did not have the energy to prepare and cook when she felt particularly low. The winter months always proved particularly difficult; in the past she managed to have her holidays in a sunny climate in November or December. Jean's depression was treated with homeopathic remedies Sepia (*see* Chapter 12) and Natrum muriaticum followed by Reiki healing (*see* Chapter 19), one-hour weekly sessions for 4 weeks. She joined a walking group and took up yoga regularly. Her condition improved markedly over the weeks and she now feels she has much more energy and can make plans for her future. Before treatment, she dreaded waking up each day wondering how she was going to cope.

Case study 4.2

Helen is a 38-year-old woman who suffered from moderate endogenous depression for a number of years. She had mixed feelings about her relationship with her partner, as there is very little physical contact. Her husband is happy with this situation. They have a 15-year-old daughter, and do not want a divorce. She also suffered from eczema, which was much worse at night in bed. Helen did not want antidepressant medication. She received homeopathic treatment, Sulphur for her eczema, Staphysagria for repressed negative feelings and emotions. Sepia was given for her mood swings. She joined a gym, because she had gained excess weight, and had Reiki healing and counselling for six sessions. Helen eventually went from working part-time to full-time employment and a change of career, which she has found much more fulfilling. She continues to have Reiki monthly on a top-up basis. The eczema has fully resolved; her resentment and mood swings are much improved.

Depression in the elderly

This condition is very common in later life and can be quite easily overlooked. This generation probably has more reasons than most to feel low. Depression presents often as a physical symptom such as tiredness, rheumatism, joint aches and pains. Sometimes it is diagnosed as dementia, because of forgetfulness or lack of memory, which can lead to confusion, loneliness, fear, and isolation. The sufferer may have lost a partner, and have no family or friends locally. Added to this is a lack of mobility, tiredness, unbalanced eating habits, sleep disturbance and lack of fresh air and exercise. These are only some of the factors that contribute to mental and emotional ill-health in the elderly, which can eventually have a negative effect and ultimately lead to low mood and depression. The quality of life is no less important at this stage of life than at any other.

Being aware of the need for diligence in detecting depression in our elderly population is paramount, according to a recent report:[5]

> When a case of depression is identified, then several principles need to be applied. Firstly, there is the need to treat the whole person including their physical and psychosocial needs. Following this, there is also the need to educate patients and carers about depression and their treatment options.

The same report concluded that:

> depression is a common condition in the elderly in hospital, existing alongside many physical conditions in a complex and interrelated way. Exact mechanisms may not be well understood at present, but proper identification and treatment of depression does have a major impact on health outcomes. It is therefore essential that all clinical staff involved in the care of older people have the requisite skills to identify and implement treatment for this condition.

A balanced diet is of the utmost importance, particularly fresh fruit and vegetables. Omega 3 and cod liver oil capsules with calcium and magnesium supplements may be considered.[6] Smaller more frequent meals for the elderly, with added vitamins plus increased fish consumption is useful for a better health balance.[7] Encouraging regular gentle exercise, where possible with fresh air, and social interaction with family and friends including local groups will help encourage mental alertness. A sense of purpose is beneficial in the course of a day or week, and may well in itself help maintain good mental health. Let us not forget that this age group deserves our care and respect; they have taught us everything we know about the human condition, we owe them a debt of gratitude.

The touch therapies are particularly useful in treating depression in the older age group, as these individuals are often deprived of this beneficial sensory stimulation.[8] Hands-on therapies help them to keep in touch with their feelings that can so easily become dissociated over a period of time particularly in isolation, and also improves emotional communication. The warmth and touch engendered by the interaction also improves relaxation, induces sleep and improves feelings of 'wellbeing'.

> A psychoneurosis must be understood, ultimately, as the suffering of a soul which has not discovered its meaning ... We cannot tolerate a lack of meaning.
>
> CG Jung[9]

References

1   Zukav G. *The Seat of the Soul*. London: Rider; 1990.
2   Ayuso-Mateos J, Vazquez-Barquero JL, Dowrick C *et al*. Depressive disorders in Europe: prevalence figures from the ODIN study. *Br J Psychiatry* 2001; 179: 308–16.
3   Singh NA and Fiatarone Singh MA. Exercise and depression in the older adult. *Nutr Clin Care* 2000; 3: 197–208.
4   Turner J, Billettt EE and Szabo A. Phenylethylamine: a possible link to the antidepressant effects of exercise. *Br J Sports Med* 2001; 35: 342–3.
5   Bullock R. Depression: pitfalls in management. *Geriatr Med* 2006; 36: 43–8.
6   Stoll AL, Severus E, Freeman M *et al*. Omega 3 fatty acids in bipolar disorders: a preliminary double-blind placebo controlled trial. *Arch Gen Psychiatry* 1999; 56: 407–12.
7   Hibbeln JR. Fish consumption and major depression. *Lancet* 1998; 35: 1213.
8   Demetriou A and Coyle M. Complementary medicine. In: Shukla RB and Brooks D (eds). *A Guide to Care of the Elderly*. London: HMSO; 1996. pp. 339–48.
9   Jung CG. *Collected Works. Volume 8*. London: Routledge Kegan Paul; 1970.

Further reading

• Atkinson S. *Climbing out of Depression*. London: Lion Publishing; 2005.
• Fennell M. *Overcoming Low Self Esteem*. London: Constable and Robinson; 2006.
• Hittleman R. *Guide to Yoga and Meditation*. New York: Bantam Books; 1981.
• Holford P. *Optimum Nutrition for the Mind*. London: Piatkus; 1998.
• Wright A. *Depression: recognition and management in general practice*. London: Royal College of General Practitioners; 1988.

Contacts

• *Alcoholics Anonymous*: tel: 0845 769 7555
• *The Association of Post Natal Illness*: www.apni.org; tel: 020 7586 0868
• *The British Association of Anger Management*: www.angermanage.co.uk; tel: 0845 1300 28
• *British SAD Association*: www.sada.org.uk; PO Box 989, Steyning PN44 3HG, UK
• *Cruse*, youth project (for individuals aged 12–18 years affected by death): www.rd4u.org.uk; helpline: 0808 808 1677
• *Manic Depression Fellowship*: www.mdf.org.uk; tel: 020 7793 2600
• *Calm* helpline for young men with depression or who are suicidal: tel: 0800 585 858
• *Mind (mental health charity)*: www.mind.org.uk; tel: 020 8519 2122
• *Samaritans*: www.samaritans.org.uk; tel: 08457 90 90 90

5

The process of death and dying

> *Death is the great wound in the universe, the root of all fear and negativity.*
> *Friendship with our death would enable us to celebrate the eternity of the soul,*
> *which death cannot touch.*
>
> *John O'Donohue[1]*

Death is the fundamental mystery of our human life cycle. It is the biggest and most profound experience through suffering and loss, and the final frontier of our physical existence. We do not prepare well for this final journey; in many respects we live in denial. Death is the only absolute certainty we have in this life.

We honour the spirit of humanity, spiritually through the symbolic ritual of the physical act of the dying and death process. This helps in many ways to heal the pain of letting go, giving a certain focus, dignity, peace of mind and often a deeper connection to the divine. Death and dying rituals are important for both the departing person and those left behind, as part of the grieving process that follows. Our greatest spiritual experiences often come through pain and suffering. We must honour and learn from this the greatest and final lesson life has to offer. We cannot avoid this finality so we might as well embrace it in all its glory.

> *I feel and know that death is not the ending as we thought, but rather the*
> *beginning – and that nothing ever is or can be lost, nor even die, nor soul, nor*
> *matter.*
>
> *Walt Whitman[2]*

Around 600 000 people die in the UK each year; of these 60% die in hospital and nursing homes, most of these are elderly, 20% die at home and 20% in a hospice environment.[3] There are 3000 hospices in the UK funded mostly by donations and supported by dedicated volunteers. If we die of cancer we will probably have what is termed a good death, with all our final needs and wishes catered for, as the standard of palliative and hospice care in the UK is excellent. The other 80% of us who do not die of cancer could find that the same standard is not universal. Good quality of care is rather like a lottery in some aspects, which vary from one end of the country to the other. In those that die suddenly, for example from heart disease, the ending here can be fairly unpredictable. Due to the advance in drug therapies, high technological surgical intervention and the very nature of the disease, terminal care is difficult to initiate. The holism of palliative care has spread, largely because of the reputation based on the hospice movement and its approach to the process of terminal care. As professional carers we can emulate this philosophy in all aspects of dying and death, both in the community and hospital settings.

The general focus of the medical profession is to prolong life by virtue of the Hippocratic oath. This is quite rightly the most ethical and moral approach to human survival. Only when life is deemed at an end can we stop looking for ways to sustain it; only then are we able to shift the focus from a living person to the dying process.

Dying and ultimate death needs are very much an individual process. For many people the ultimate would be to die suddenly without pain or knowing, for others it would be the freedom of symptoms of the dying process, pain and anxiety and being able to choose where to die: at home, in hospital or in a hospice setting. People who live by cultural and religious faiths may want to experience dying as a physical phenomenon and in a state of spiritual connectedness to the divine. In this state, death is not deemed a failure but more an expectation in life and a renewal or rebirth in the next life.

Dying and death can engender absolute terror into our very heart and soul, and to some degree this is present in everyone. The termination of our existence and the acceptance of our finality, the giving up our future, have to be embraced in all their aspects and this cannot be achieved without anxiety, pain and a lot of soul searching. Because life, despite all its failings, is deemed a great and precious gift, we do not let it go lightly.

Caring for the dying can become the deepest experience of love and humility; this process of the ending of life has a mutual dependence. The need for love and support is greater than ever in order for both the living and dying to let go and bear witness to the ending process. Dying should not be left to our professional caring services; we are all involved at a human level and need the emotional experience for future reference. In many ways it is the reason we have lived; as we celebrate life, so too the death of that life, our cycle of birth, life and death is complete. A good and loving death gives us the opportunity to connect to the divine within all of us. As we become familiar with this process, it will help dispel the mystery of dying and the fear that it brings, and will make the inevitable easier to accept.

On the debate of assisted dying and euthanasia, in the UK the Royal College of Physicians and the Royal College of General Practitioners concluded that properly funded and accessible palliative care services are essential for meeting the needs of those with terminal illness. They have urged the government to recognise the need for greater funding for palliative care and to acknowledge that palliative care is a major part of the NHS end-of-life programmes, such as the Liverpool Care Pathway for the Dying. They also recognise that reliable provision of end-of-life care for the elderly is a challenge yet to be met.[4]

> *Come to me all who are weary and find life burdensome and I will refresh you. Take my yoke upon your shoulders and learn from me, for I am gentle and humble of heart. Your souls will find rest, for my yoke is easy and my burden light.*
>
> *Matthew 11:28–30*

An awareness and knowledge of cultural and religious observances

It is extremely important that as a diverse cultural nation we embrace all aspects of religious and spiritual needs, particularly in the process of death and dying. The following are some of the cultural and religious faiths we need to be aware of. For staff caring for the dying, it is important to realise that the rituals observed are not a morbid obsession, but a key part of religious faith.[5,6]

Christianity

Catholics and Orthodox Christians expect a priest to give them final confession, holy communion and anoint them with oil. Prayer is a major part of a Christian death. In Ireland, both Catholic and Protestants place great importance on services before death, followed by a wake (watch) and a large community funeral.

Church of England

The process in the Church of England is very similar in principle to other Christian faiths but has less ceremonial content and there is usually no formal ritual of after care. The dying process tends to be very reserved, a quiet, dignified and fairly solemn affair.

Christian Scientist and Seventh Day Adventist

Members of these religions will not necessarily always have conventional treatment and will have variations in needs as Christians in terms of symbolic themes and rites of the dying process. Church elders will often advise on what is helpful and necessary for them.

Black African and Pentacostalist

The basic health care is the same as for Christians. The dead person is never left alone, to prevent spirits from invading the body. This is deemed a joyful occasion, with deliberate wailing and crying rituals and performances, which continues for a set period of mourning.

Judaism

Jews have a firm belief in an afterlife, the same as Christians. There are dietary needs, for example kosher food (meat that has been killed according to Jewish law), no pork, shellfish and no mixing of meat and milk. Burial takes place within 48 hours of dying. The deceased is not left alone until burial takes place, as a mark of respect. Unless permission is given, staff cannot lay out the body.

Jehovah's Witness

The most important part of a Jehovah's Witness' life and death is the very strict adherence to their rule of not having blood transfusions or blood products to enhance or save life. Otherwise their holistic care is the same as for Christians.

Islam

Muslims pray five times a day, facing Mecca. The dying do not have to observe Ramadan (month's fast); at this stage it is their choice. No alcohol is allowed (some drug cocktails include alcohol), and strict diet is observed with no pork or pork products. Muslims tend to eat a vegetarian diet in hospital/hospices. A dying person is faced towards Mecca and prayers are said with the family and the community. Only Muslims can touch the body in death. It is important that rubber gloves are worn by carers who are not Muslim, when handling the body. The remains are buried facing Mecca and are never cremated. The Muslim community will advise on basic needs and rites of passage. Funeral arrangements are made within 48 hours.

Hinduism

This religion incorporates many gods and goddesses, but they are a manifestation of the one God. Hindus believe the dead return to earth in a different form. No anger is expressed in physical dying, as death and rebirth are readily accepted. Ashes are usually returned to the Ganges, which is their spiritual home. Prayer and spiritual awareness are the most important factors. A diet of beef or its products is forbidden, as the cow is deemed a sacred animal. The Hindu community is happy to advise on specific needs of the dying.[6]

Sikhism

Members of the Sikh community have symbols of uncut hair covered by a turban for both men and women. The dead are usually cremated, and the ashes taken to India and scattered in the Punjab, the birthplace of Sikhism. Shorts or underpants of the dying are never removed (the individual always has to have a leg in one to change to another pair of shorts or underpants). Hair loss through chemotherapy can be very distressing, the remaining hair can be secured by the use of a hair net. There is generally a large number of family and friends present with the dying person. A separate room away from busy wards is ideal for grieving families. The Sikh community likes to keep symbols next to the dying body, for example steel bangles or small daggers. Rituals and rites are all community based.[6]

Buddhism

This is not a religion as such, more of a way of life based on meditation in order to reach Nirvana. The Dalai Lama is the spiritual head. The body is believed to be a temporary vessel for supporting spiritual life. Buddhists aspire to as near perfect a death as possible in a calm experiencing state without conventional help. Buddhists may well not want intervention, such as medication for pain relief, as this is deemed a failure or a weakening of the spirit. Their dietary needs are usually vegetarian.

Chinese

The Chinese may be Christian or Buddhist with cultural differences, a belief in the afterlife and worship of ancestors. It is family and community orientated and also includes prayers and offerings to the spirits of the dead ancestors. Altars are built for the spirits as part of the dying process. The coffin quite often resides in the dying person's room. A member of the clergy, or a Buddhist brother or sister usually visits with the dying person and their family. Basic nursing care needs are often carried out by family and friends. Incense and firecrackers are sometimes used to ward off evil spirits. The body will often be dressed in robes like those of a Buddhist priest. Ritual means everything to the family and community. The family and Chinese community will advise on what is appropriate for them.[5]

Helpful information for the dying process

The transition from life to death is made much easier if information and communication are readily available between the dying person, their family and the professionals who are caring for them. The first priority is to establish where and how the dying person would like to end their days. A medical and nursing assessment is then carried out.

Cultural awareness

The dying person will be reassured and more relaxed if their last rites and needs are met. They can die in dignity, according to their cultural or religious heritage and beliefs.

Information and communication

In many instances where the person is unable to communicate their needs with the staff, family and friends should be consulted instead. If there is a language communication problem then the use of an interpreter friend or family member is invaluable. The family should be informed regularly of any change in the dying person's condition. During physical care routines it is important to make sure that the dying person is informed of procedures and treatments. Members of the family and community are only too willing to explain rituals, needs and cultural nuances. Communication is also important, with the many other visiting professional bodies, for example the clergy, counsellors, physical therapists and teachers, particularly if a child is dying. Feelings and emotions of loved ones are unpredictable at this time – fear, shock and disbelief are all valid emotions. In a busy hospital setting, a quiet room is more appropriate to allow the family to stay with the dying person to the end.

Dignity

The dying person should be handled physically and emotionally with great respect and dignity whatever their background or cultural needs. Avoid overcrowding in a small room with a constant stream of visitors, as the patient can become overwhelmed and anxious. A constant acknowledgement of visitors can be a great strain on the patient and the family.

Physical needs

Some families and communities express a wish to help with the physical and practical needs of the dying person, and want to be close to them for as long as possible. They should be encouraged to participate fully as this will help them with the grieving process that follows.

Unfinished business

If possible it is useful as part of the end-of-life process to help sort out wills, put affairs in order and say goodbyes. Informing family members that the patient may have lost touch with helps to alleviate anxiety, and allows a more peaceful death.

Home care

This follows the same principle as the care in the hospice movement, with family, doctor, clergy, Macmillan and district nurses in attendance. The family is still in control of basic needs, which will help with anxiety on both sides and makes the subsequent bereavement much more tangible.

Emotions of the caregivers

It is extremely valuable for nurses, doctors and other carers to acknowledge their own feelings of grief and loss. In order to tend the needs of the dying, we become attached emotionally, particularly if it is over a long period of time, or if a child is involved. It is a natural human emotion and there is no loss of professionalism in an appropriate grief reaction. In some cases, attending the funeral helps the professionals and the family to deal with their emotions and feelings.

A designated care team

This is the most important time of our life. It is the stage of giving up the future. It is very upsetting if the dying and their family do not know which members of the caring professions to approach to ask for help.

No one should die alone

St John of the Cross:

> *In order to experience pleasure in all (todo)*
> *Desire to have pleasure in nothing (nada)*
> *In order to arrive at possessing all,*
> *Desire to possess nothing,*
> *In order to arrive at being all,*
> *Desire to be nothing,*
> *In order to arrive at knowing all,*
> *Desire to know nothing.*

> *The Ascent of Mount Carmel, 1,13,11*

Complementary therapies and dying

Apart from nursing care and analgesic drugs necessary for pain relief, complementary therapies help to relieve the discomfort, aid sleep and help calm and relax the system of the dying person. The hands-on gentle therapies are beneficial and recommended for the end-of-life care. Refer to Chapter 29, Palliative care (p. 177).

Massage

This is a gentle hands-on touch technique, which will help relieve aches and pains allowing the patient to relax and feel more comfortable (*see* Chapter 14). Most of all, it is of a great emotional comfort, communicating loving care.

Aromatherapy

A relaxing gentle massage with fragrant oils will heighten the senses and will help to induce sleep and a feeling of 'wellbeing' (*see* Chapter 8).

Reflexology

A foot massage stimulates many different parts of the body to induce a 'feel good factor' and relieve pain. It may also induce calmer breathing at the end of life (*see* Chapter 18).

Homeopathic remedies beneficial for end-of-life care

- *Arsenicum*: to help calm fear and restlessness
- *Aconite napellis*: this is useful for acute fear
- *Arnica*: for aches and pains
- *Gelsemium*: to induce relaxation
- *Natrum muriaticum*: for sadness and tearfulness
- *Avena sativa*: this tincture can be used to help induce relaxation and promote sleep

Prayer and meditation

These are useful as therapies as well as cultural needs to help with fear and anxiety of parting, and can become for some an integral part of the end-of-life process (*see* Chapters 15 and 17).

> *When the earth shall claim your limbs then shall you truly dance.*
>
> *Kahlil Gibran*[7]

References

1 O'Donohue J. *Anam Cara. Spiritual Wisdom from the Celtic World.* London: Bantam Press; 1999.
2 Whitman W. *Prose Works.* Philadelphia, PA: David Mackey; 1892.
3 Denis T and Rooney C. Office for National Statistics. *Health Stat Q* 1999; 1: 1–3.
4 Boyle A. Assisted dying: is better palliative care the answer. *Geriatr Med* 2006; 36: 9–11.

5   Neuberger J. *Caring for Dying People of Different Faiths*. Oxford: Radcliffe Publishing; 2004.
6   Henley A. *Asians in Britain* (3 volumes): *Caring for Sikhs and their Families: religious aspects of care; Caring for Muslims and their Families: religious aspects of care; Caring for Hindus and their Families: religious aspects of care*. DHSS and King Edward's Hospital Fund for London: National Extension College; 1982–84.
7   Gibran K. *The Prophet*. Middlesex: Penguin Books; 1992.

Further reading

- Bernardin Cardinal J. *The Gift of Peace*. London: Darton Longman and Todd; 1998.
- Black D. *When Patients Die: learning to live with the loss of a patient*. London: Routledge; 2003.
- Cobb M and Robshaw V (eds). *The Spiritual Challenge of Healthcare*. Edinburgh: Churchill Livingstone; 1998.
- Kubler Ross E. *On Death and Dying*. London: Tavistock; 1970.
- Kubler Ross E. *On Children and Death*. London. Touchstone Books; 1997.
- Kubler Ross E. *To Live until we say Goodbye*. London: Touchstone Books; 1997.
- Kubler Ross E. *On Life after Death*. London: Celestial Arts; 1991.
- Neuberger J. *Dying Well, a Guide to Enabling a Good Death*. Oxford: Radcliffe Publishing; 2004.
- Nouwen HJM. *Our Greatest Gift. A meditation on dying and caring*. London: Hodder and Stoughton Publishers; 1994.
- Sanders C, Summers DH and Tellor N. *Hospice: the living idea*. London: Edward Arnold; 1981.
- Waterhouse M. *Staying Close: a positive approach to dying and bereavement*. London: Constable; 2003.

Contacts

- *British Heart Foundation*: www.bhf.org.uk; information line: 08450 708070
- *The Buddhist Hospice Trust*: www.buddhisthospice.org.uk
- *Cancer Help*: www.cancerhelp.org.uk
- *Child Death Helpline*: Bereavement Services Department, Great Ormond St. Hospital NHS Trust, Great Ormond Street, London WC1N 3JH; tel: 020 7813 8551; helpline 0800282986
- *The Cicely Saunders Foundation*: www.cicelysaundersfoundation.org
- *The Compassionate Friends*: 53 North Street, Bristol B53 1EN; tel: 0117 966 5252; helpline: 0117 953 9639
- *Cruse Bereavement Care*: Cruse House, 126 Shoa Road, Richmond, Surrey TW9 1UR; tel: 020 8940 481
- *The Iain Rennie Hospice at Home*: www.irhh.org; tel: 01422 890222
- *King's College London, Department of Palliative Care*: www.kclac.uk/palliative
- *Macmillan Cancer Support*: 89 Albert Embankment, London SE1 7UQ; tel: 020 7840 7840; information line: 0845 601 6161; www.macmillan.org.uk
- *National Council for Hospices and Specialist Palliative Care Services*: 34–44 Britannia Street, London WC1X 9JG; tel: 020 7520 8299
- *The Natural Death Centre*: www.naturaldeath.org.uk; 6 Blackstock Mews, Blackstock Road, London N4 2BT; tel: 020 7359 8391; email: rhiao@dial.pipex.com

6

Bereavement

The experience of one's own truth ... makes it possible to return to one's world of feeling at an adult level without paradise, but with the ability to mourn.

Alice Miller[1]

Bereavement is the process that includes grief and mourning. Grief is a normal reaction to intense sorrow over the loss of a significant person, or object, or part of the self, or of a previous stage of the life cycle. Death of course is not the only loss we need to mourn, although it is likely to be the greatest. Women who have experienced a miscarriage, stillbirth, hysterectomy or mastectomy also need to grieve. The loss of independence, through chronic disease, redundancy, being uprooted from one country to another, or even the death of a treasured pet needs to go through the grieving process. All loss requires a period of mourning and adjustment. Otherwise, as our biography is our biology (our emotional and psychological history is imprinted in the physical) there is a danger that long-term health problems will ensue.[2] In many respects we have been programmed to deal with loss from an early age because we go through many difficult stages and changes in our lifetime. Hopefully in time we will have gained the emotional skill and experience to deal with greater loss.

Our greatest suffering comes from the death of someone we love. The loss of adult loved ones in our society is difficult to come to terms with, but the death of a beloved child is even more bewildering and traumatic and for some it can take a lifetime to recover. Death is an experience society does not want to acknowledge, almost to the point of 'if we don't talk about it or entertain the idea it won't happen to me', which leaves us unprepared, particularly on an emotional level. Death is seldom talked about and rarely witnessed these days. Our elderly and terminally ill are admitted to hospitals, hospices, and nursing homes. The ending of life to ultimate death can be very institutionalised and clinical, so we are gradually seeing less of the human process of dying. This lack of witnessing and contact can make dying and death a very frightening experience. The hospice movement goes some way to redressing the balance, where families are encouraged to take part in the ending of a loved one's life and to bear witness to that ending. This helps to demystify and 'normalise' death as a healthy process of our life cycle, creating an acceptance. Spiritual belief has a major influence in resolving the grief earlier than in people who have no spiritual belief.[3]

Pathological grief is more likely to occur following:

- the loss of a child
- sudden or violent death, e.g. accident, murder or suicide
- lack of emotional support
- lack of normal coping strategies
- bad experience of loss or separation in childhood

- mental health problems
- a multiple or major loss over a short period of time.

The stages of grief

The emotional journey of grief and mourning has four main stages:

1 shock
2 anger
3 sadness
4 acceptance.

Feelings associated with these stages, for practical purposes, are discussed below.

Shock

- *Numbness*: it's like a bad dream. It takes a while to sink in
- *Helplessness*: expressing profound feelings of powerlessness and fear of being left alone
- *Fear* of an emotional breakdown and that someone else will die
- *Longing*: for all that is lost and that life will never be the same again

Anger

- Examples of this are 'why me' anger at society, at doctors and perhaps at lack of support
- *Guilt*: for being alive, things not said and often for not coping

Sadness

- For a future without them, memories of the past, dreams about the person that died and the ending of life
- *Physical symptoms*: insomnia, loss of appetite, exhaustion, being accident prone, and difficulty in concentration and focusing

Acceptance

This phase can take at least 1 to 2 years depending on the circumstances of the death and recovery process and survival abilities of the grieving family. If it is a child that dies, the process can take much longer. Then follows the rebuilding of a life and future without the loved one.

The stages of grief do not necessary follow in any particular order or time scale; these are a guide only.

Affection shown by a gentle touch can still a troubled mind.

Betty Shine[4]

Children in the grieving process

- A child's feelings should be acknowledged.
- Adults must pay attention and show an interest in normal daily events.
- Children express themselves better by drawing and acting out feeling events.
- Children can show great distress one minute and are fine the next.
- It helps if children are part of the services and if possible see the body and say goodbye.
- School should be informed.
- It is important to return to the routine of home and school life as soon as possible.
- Adults worry about the unpredictable behaviour of children following a loss.
- Children should be encouraged to talk about the person that died.
- Children should witness adults in tears to know that it is normal.
- It is important to reinforce that the death is not their fault.

Managing the grieving process

The conventional medical approach is, as a general rule, often in the form of hypnotics and/or tranquillisers, which can be of use for a short time, for some. There are no shortcuts with grief, it tends to be a fairly long slow process with a steep learning curve on survival skills. We must accept that grief following the loss of someone significant is normal and painful. Any attempt, with whatever therapy, to avoid or deny the process of mourning is bound to result in long-term health problems.

Bereavement counselling

- If appropriate, most hospices do provide counselling and support services.
- In many areas there are also voluntary and local community counselling services.
- There is no substitute for vocal expression of grief and the need to repeat the event is compelling. **Feelings of grief** have to be **heard, acknowledged and understood** so that it can be emotionally processed.

Homoeopathy

Suggested remedies include:

- *Avena sativa*: to induce relaxation and sleep
- *Aconite napellis, Arnica*: in a case of shock
- *Ignatia*: for unpredictable emotions
- *Nux vomica*: for anger and resentment
- *Natrum muriaticum*: for tearfulness

Massage

When we lose someone close we miss the physical touch and the comfort that it brings. Massage also has a relaxation and calming effect and will help to induce sleep (*see* Chapter 14).

Reiki

This form of energy healing will balance negative emotions and help to restore perspective and logic, with a relaxation and calming effect on the system (*see* Chapter 19).

Diet

Lack of interest in food is quite common. Eating smaller meals more often and adding extra fresh fruit and vegetables can help restore a more normal balance. Increasing the intake of water and fresh fruit juice is also recommended because the system can become quite sluggish at this time. Avoidance or reduction of coffee and alcohol will help, as these are stimulants and will prevent refreshing sleep (*see* Chapter 22).

Self-help

The mind, body and spirit need regular nourishment to ensure development and growth. At times of grief it is difficult to make sense of life events. To have someone or a place to turn to for support is important, for example **a close friend, family or agency, places of worship/organised religion such as churches, synagogues, mosques.**

In times of need, prayers, meditation, bereavement support and practical community help are often readily available. Sharing experiences of loss with those with similar needs is beneficial for recovery. Long-term interests are also important for life in the future and as a means of maintaining human contact.

Pets

Treasured family pets give a great deal of comfort and help with loneliness and isolation. This is particularly the case with older people who are left to grieve on their own following the death of a spouse.

How to help people grieve following a significant loss

DO ...

- show your genuine *concern and caring*
- be available to *listen/help* with whatever else seems needed at the time
- say you are *sorry* about what happened and acknowledge their pain
- allow them to *express as much unhappiness as they are feeling* and wish to share with you
- encourage them to *be patient with their progress*, not to expect too much too soon
- allow them to *talk* about their loss as much and as often as they want
- *talk about the special endearing qualities* of that person they've lost
- reassure, that *they did everything they could.*

DON'T ...

- let your own sense of helplessness keep you from reaching out
- avoid them because of your own discomfort. Being avoided by friends adds pain to an already painful experience
- say you know how they feel
- tell them what they should feel or do or think
- change the subject when they talk about their loss
- avoid mentioning their loss in case it reminds them of their pain. They have not forgotten it
- try to find a positive aspect about the loss (a moral lesson, closer family ties)
- point out at least they have their other ...
- say they can always have another ...
- suggest they be grateful for ...
- make any comments that in any way suggest their loss was their fault. There will be enough feelings of doubt and guilt already.

Case study 6.1: An Irish wake – a bereavement process

Kathleen Coyle at 87 led a full life. A mother of 11 children, five born at the family home and six were born in the local hospital. Living in the Donegal countryside just over the border from Derry, her home was the 'crossroads' for all her family. Sadly, she developed congestive cardiac failure and died a week later in the local hospital in Letterkenny.

What an occasion
For two days and two nights following her death her wake took place. The priest initiated prayers at the start of this period. Not only the family but hundreds of neighbours and friends came to pay their respects. She was taken from the hospital to her home where for the two days a continuous stream of visitors came from far and wide. Even the postman came to pay his respects. Not only had he delivered her post, but he had also read out the postcards to her when her vision started to deteriorate in her latter years. This was real community in mourning. Hundreds of people came with genuine sympathy for the family in mourning, and with their own personal feelings of community loss they visited Kathleen in her home. Each person visited her room, where the open coffin lay. They blessed themselves, and a prayer or two later they emerged from her room into the living room to be met by more family with offerings of tea and sandwiches. The family 'accompanied' Kathleen throughout the day and night during the wake.

In the evenings everyone took part in the Rosary, where prayers are repeated over and over again with the help of the Rosary beads. This process was a celebration of her life, as part of the Irish Catholic tradition, a thanksgiving by all the family and the community.

The whole family had a role in arranging the funeral. Everyone seemed to know what to do. Decisions on readings, flowers and church arrangements all seemed to 'flow'. The family took it in turns to keep awake so that in death Kathleen would not be left alone. There was no end to the continuous stream of refreshments from the kitchen, helped by the whole community.

The hugs and the handshakes were heartfelt. Death is part of life in Ireland. Acceptance of 'God's will' comes readily. The reason for this is that families talk about the process of death before someone dies, which brings death into the perspective of everyday existence.

The whole house was buzzing with life during the wake. Happy memories were discussed. Kathleen's husband William had died 23 years earlier. Margaret, one of her daughters, had also died 11 years before, so they both came into the community and family discussions. Happy 'banter' stories, happenings and *endings*.

On the Friday morning one hour before the funeral Mass at the local church St Baithin's in the village, the hearse arrives.

With prayers in progress the coffin lid is sealed. The sons and grandsons take it in turns in groups to carry her coffin for several hundred yards towards the village before making her final journey in the hearse to the local Catholic church.

She is carried into the chapel to the sound of 'Here I am Lord' on the violin played by her grandson, Chris. During the funeral Mass, the church is completely full and many mourners are now standing outside. During communion more music is played on the violin. The final journey is accompanied by 'I'll take you home again Kathleen' followed by 'Danny boy' before she is taken to her final resting place to be buried next to her husband, William.

The 500 or so mourners then meet for refreshments in the resource centre situated near the church. The usual exchanges take place, but there is an air of optimism about the whole process of a wake and the funeral. Of course it is sad, but it's a 'positive' sadness. This was a true celebration of a long and productive life.

In the evening a meal is arranged in a local hotel for 80 family members, where Kathleen's life continued to be celebrated.

This is a demonstration of the togetherness of a family in grief as there is in any culture, in any part of the world. What is a potentially sad affair turns out to be a very dignified, religious, family and community process where emotional and practical support is in abundance: true caring, true kindness and heartfelt sympathy.

What is different is the time it takes for a wake to 'process' those feelings and needs of the family and the community. Unhurried, this gives the opportunity for the grieving to begin. It felt as if Kathleen was part of the wake, not as a dead person but still very much alive in 'the transitory' phase of life and death. Yet, death is final. The wake ensured an opportunity for a proper 'goodbye' and a reminder that we will meet again, the Catholic belief in life after death.

How we deal with our grief depends on many factors, but an Irish wake illustrates one way to help our grieving process as part of normal life.

> *Death is only an horizon and an horizon is only the limit of our sight.*
> *Henry Scott Holland*[5]

References

1 Miller A. *The Drama of the Gifted Child. The Search for the True Self.* New York: HarperCollins; 1981.
2 Myss C. *Sacred Contracts. Awakening your divine potential.* London: Bantam Books; 2001.
3 Walsh K, King, M, Jones L *et al.* Spiritual beliefs may affect outcome of bereavement: prospective study. *BMJ* 2002; 324: 1551.
4 Shine B. *A Mind of Your Own.* London: HarperCollins; 1998.
5 Holland HS. *Death is Only an Horizon.* Hampshire: Redemptorist Publications; 1989.

Further reading

- Baglou L. *Contemporary Christian Counselling.* Sydney: EJ Dwyer; 1996.
- Bernadin J. *The Gift of Peace.* London: Darton-Longman and Todd; 1998.
- Black D. *When Patients Die: learning to live with a loss of a patient.* London: Routledge; 1999.
- Duffy W. *Children and Bereavement.* London: National Society/Church House Publishing; 1995.
- Kubler-Ross E. *On Death and Dying.* London: Simon and Schuster; 1987.
- O' Reilly P. *Dying with Love.* Dublin: Veritas; 1992.
- O'Donohue J. *ANAM CARA Spiritual Wisdom From The Celtic World.* London: Bantam Press; 1997.
- Powell J. *Abortion – the Silent Holocaust.* London: Argue Communications; 1981.
- Simpson R. *Before We Say Goodbye.* London: HarperCollins Publishers; 2001.
- Waterhouse M. *Staying Close: a positive approach to dying and bereavement.* London: Constable; 2003.

Contacts

- *Age Concern*: Astral House, 268 London Rd, London SW16 4ER; tel: 020 8765 7200
- *Citizens Advice Bureau*: www.citizensadvice.org.uk
- *Cruse* (bereavement care): www.crusebereavementcare.org.uk; CRUSE House, 126 Sheen Rd, Richmond, Surrey TW9 1UR; tel: 020 8939 9530; helpline: 0870 167 1677
- *Compassionate Friends* (international organisation) for bereaved parents: 53 North St, Bristol B53 1EM; tel: 0117 966 5202; helpline: 0117 953 9639
- *Help The Aged*: 207–221 Pentonville Rd, London N1 9UZ; tel: 020 7278 1114
- *Local Benefits Agency*: www.direct.gov.uk/mycouncil
- *The Samaritans*: www.samaritans.org.uk; helpline: 08457 90 90 90
- *SANDS*: Stillbirth and Neonatal Death Society, 28 Portland Place, London W18 1LY; tel: 020 7436 5881
- *Scotland Concern*: 113 Rose St, Edinburgh EH2 3DT; tel: 0131 220 3345
- *Victim Support*: www.victimsupport.org.uk; helpline: 0845 30 30 900

Therapies, health and lifestyle

7

Acupuncture

The soul as temple of memory: the Celtic stories suggest that time as the rhythm of soul has an eternal dimension where everything is gathered and minded. Here nothing is lost.

John O'Donohue[1]

Acupuncture has been an integral part of traditional Chinese medicine (TCM) for more than 2000 years. It is a concept of the Taoist philosophy. This is based on a belief that the human body is in a state of dynamic interaction with nature, environment and universe. It is still part of routine medical training in China. Acupuncture is one of the main approaches of Chinese medicine and the most thoroughly researched and documented of all the complementary therapies. In addition to treating specific problems, it is also deemed to have a supporting and stimulating effect on the immune system and to improve the circulation.[2,3] It may also be used to stimulate hormones, which help the body respond more efficiently to stress or injury.[3]

Acupuncture is widely accepted as an integrated holistic therapeutic tool used to complement healthcare services in the NHS. It is used extensively in palliative care, pain clinics, in primary care, physiotherapy departments and in private clinics throughout the country. Many doctors, nurses and midwives practise acupuncture as part of their routine healthcare work.

There are many types of acupuncture practised in the west, but the most commonly used is the Chinese traditional method. An experienced acupuncturist will do a thorough examination of the body and decide which points or appropriate meridians (*see* below) require treatment.

History, philosophy and evidence

The Chinese medical philosophy is concerned with balance, between two naturally opposing forces, for example *yin* (dark, passive and tranquil female energy) and *yang* (light, male aggressive and stimulating energy) in a healthy functioning body. This includes balancing heat, cold, internal and external, excess and deficiency and also assessing and responding to the cyclical effects of the five elements, *water, fire, earth, wood* and *metal*. This effect can be felt physically and emotionally at different times throughout the year.

According to this theory, the life energy that surrounds the body in general flows through the system and is called *qi* (pronounced 'chee'). Many factors can disturb or disrupt this energy flow – psychological problems, physical illness or environmental factors. The energy can become blocked, or can flow too fast, or too slowly, creating an imbalance eventually causing ill-health. To prevent this from happening and to restore good health, *qi* will be brought back into balance, using the traditional Chinese methods of acupuncture.

In Chinese medicine, the body is divided into 12 main pathways, or energy channels, known as *meridians*. Each meridian is linked to a particular organ in the body, and each organ can be treated by stimulating the relevant meridian. There are more than 2000 acupuncture points on the surface of the body, but around 365 are used in everyday practice. An acupuncturist using very fine needles will activate or unblock these energy channels in order to treat and prevent disease, boost the body's natural healing immune system, alleviate pain, relieve fatigue and promote relaxation, resulting in a feeling of 'wellbeing'.

The British Medical Acupuncture Society (BMAS) is a nationwide group of family doctors and hospital specialists who practise acupuncture integrated with mainstream medicine. The BMAS believes that while it is exciting that the range of medical applications of acupuncture is increasing, it does mean that the responsible practitioner of acupuncture has a duty to educate both other medical colleagues and the general public about the strengths and weaknesses of the technique. The ideal promoted by the BMAS is that acupuncture should be fully incorporated or integrated into orthodox medicine and used as one of the therapeutic tools available in treatment of a defined range of conditions. Clearly, a GP or hospital doctor who is trained in the use of acupuncture can do this, but safe and considered therapy may be available from a non-medical practitioner who works in close communication and co-operation with a patient's doctor.[2]

Most of the scientific studies on acupuncture have been on the analgesic aspects of pain relief. Acupuncture is effective in treating pain; it works 70–80% of the time, far more than the placebo effect, which has around 30% efficacy.[3] Veterinary surgeons in China have used acupuncture to treat animals successfully.[3]

This meridian system of acupuncture was established by French researcher Pierre de Vernejoul. He injected radioactive isotopes into the acupoints of humans and tracked their movements with a gamma-imaging camera. The isotopes travelled 30 cm along acupuncture meridians within 4–6 minutes. Vernejoul then challenged his own work by injecting isotopes into the blood vessels at random areas of the body rather than into acupoints. The isotopes did not travel in the same way, further indicating that the meridians do indeed comprise a system of separate pathways within the body.[4,5]

Neurological research in the late 1970s discovered the naturally occurring chemicals in the body known as endorphins.[3] By binding to the opiate receptors that are found throughout the nervous system, endorphins are able to block pain. The hypothalamus–pituitary releases beta-endorphins into the blood and cerebral spinal fluid to create an analgesic effect, inhibiting brain signals. Dr Bruce Pomeranz discovered that pretreating rats with the drug naloxone, which is known to block healing endorphins, could not achieve acupuncture pain relief. This finding suggested that endorphins released by acupuncture stimulus were an important mechanism in the pain-relieving effect of acupuncture.[3] Pomeranz subsequently studied the effect of electrical stimulation and manipulation of the needles. He discovered the difference between high-frequency, low-intensity and low-frequency, high-intensity stimulation. The low-frequency, high-intensity stimulation produced an analgesic effect that was slower at the beginning, longer in duration and also with an accumulative effect. The high-frequency, low-intensity stimulation produced rapid analgesic effects, very effective for acute pain, and was shorter in duration, with no accumulative effect.[3]

Applications in modern medicine

Conditions suitable for acupuncture include:

- allergies, allergic rhinitis, hay fever, urticaria
- mild incontinence
- irritable bowel syndrome
- migraines, headaches
- smoking cessation
- musculoskeletal pain
- menopausal, menstrual and premenstrual problems
- sinus problems, chronic catarrh
- sports injuries, neuralgias, muscle strains
- fibromyalgia
- general pain relief
- palliative care.

Practical points in acupuncture

Fine needles, usually disposable sterile needles, are inserted, which is normally a very quick, painless, bloodless procedure. The needles are usually rotated between finger and thumb to 'draw or disperse energy' from a point of a meridian. The patient feels slight numbness or a tingling sensation over each point. The needles penetrate the skin and are inserted a quarter to half an inch in depth. The number of needles used varies from one to as many as 15 at any one time. Generally, the more experienced the therapist the fewer needles used. They may be left in for a few minutes or for up to half an hour depending on the patient's needs, reactions and the condition that is being treated.

> *A loving heart is the truest wisdom.*
>
> *Charles Dickens[6]*

References

1 O'Donohue J. *Anam Cara. Spiritual Wisdom from the Celtic World*. London: Bantam Press; 1999.
2 The British Medical Acupuncture Society BMAS. www.medical-acupuncture.co.uk (accessed 10 October 2006).
3 Stux G and Pomeranz B. *Acupuncture: a textbook and atlas*. Berlin: Springer-Verlag; 1987.
4 Gerber R. *Vibrational Medicine for the 21st Century*. New York: Eagle Brook; 2000.
5 Darras JC, de Vernejoul P, Albarede P *et al*. Nuclear medicine investigation of transmission of acupuncture information. *Acupunct Med* 1993; 11: 22–8.
6 Dickens C. *David Copperfield*. Oxford: Oxford University Press; 1981.

Further reading

- Ceniceros S and Brown GR. Acupuncture: A review of its history, theories and indications. *South Med J* 1998; 91: 1121–5.
- Fulder S. *The Handbook of Complementary Medicine*. London: Century; 1989.
- Lewith G. *Acupuncture – Its Place in Medical Science*. London: Merlin; 1989.

- Shapiro D. *Your Body Speaks Your Mind*. London: Piatkus; 1997.
- Thomas K, Nicholl JP and Fall M. Access to complementary health care via general practice. *Br J Gen Pract* 2001; 51: 25–30.

Contacts

- *British Acupuncture Council and Register*: www.acupuncture.org.uk; Park House, 63 Jeddo Road, London W12 9HQ; tel: 020 8735 0400
- *British Medical Acupuncture Society* (BMAS): www.medical-acupuncture.org.uk; 12 Marbury House, Higher Whitley, Warrington, Cheshire WA4 4QW; tel: 01925 730727

8

Aromatherapy

Faith is being sure what we hope for and certain of what we do not see.
Hebrews 11:1

Aromatherapy is a holistic treatment using the hands to massage essential oils, which are extracted from plants, onto the surface of the body. This therapy is used to enhance a feeling of 'wellbeing' and promote emotional and physical good health. It is used for a wide variety of complaints, but most commonly as a treatment to relieve musculoskeletal conditions and symptoms of stress, anxiety and depression. Much of the aromatherapy work in the past was practised in beauty salons, sports facilities, health clubs, gyms and private clinics. It has now become firmly integrated with our therapeutic healthcare system and more recently in primary care, hospitals, palliative care and hospices.

Aroma (aromatic or scent) therapy (healing) combines touch with aromatic oils. This is a simple and natural way to convey healing. In so doing it stimulates, vitalises, soothes, stretches and relaxes the mind and body, thus combining the two most powerful senses of touch and smell. These oils can also be used in other ways to promote healing apart from massage, for example in bath water and as a compress or inhalation.

Humans have a highly developed sense of touch and smell, with instant effects promoting lasting benefits. Mothers and babies bond using these finely honed nurturing senses. Lovers are attracted to each other by naturally secreted hormones (pheromones). Smell can be mood changing or enhancing and can be effective in pain relief. Substantial evidence exists that odours can have a positive effect on mood. As early as 1908 Freud stressed the importance of olfaction and emotion in his description of a patient with an obsessional neurosis.[1] Studies also suggest that individuals in a positive state of mind are less affected by pain or stress and are more focused on their recovery.[1]

History, philosophy and evidence

Aromatherapy as a holistic and therapeutic aid has been used for around 5000 years. The ancient Egyptians are thought to have pioneered aromatics, and became experts through studies of plants and herbs.[2] They used them extensively for medicinal purposes for cosmetics use, religious ceremonies (incense) and the embalming of dead bodies. This was used as an antiseptic to protect and preserve the Egyptian body in its tomb, ensuring its safe journey to the 'next life'. Myrrh and cedar wood were found on bandages of 'mummies' excavated from ancient Egyptian archaeological sites; these had properties that slowed down the decomposition of the body. The pharaohs were also known to use poppy seeds and extracts to help calm fractious children during times of illness.

The ancient Greeks gained their knowledge and skills from the Egyptians. They then explored it further and realised that certain odours or fragrances from flowers and herbs had different effects, some with stimulating and others with relaxing properties. Early in the evolution of aromatherapy, oils were used to absorb the fragrances from the plants, herbs and flowers that were used in cosmetics and for medicinal purposes. Greek soldiers used myrrh in ointments to treat wounds. Hippocrates the Greek physician in the 4th century BC used frankincense, rose of opium and myrrh to help eradicate the smell of the plague from Athens. He advocated 'The way to health is to have an aromatic bath and scented massage every day'. The Romans gathered their wisdom of aromatics from Greek doctors who worked in Rome at that time. They also used them as personal beauty treatments, bathing oils and perfumes. Damascus in Syria became a major rose producer in the 14th century. Then between the 14th and 17th centuries Europe was in the middle of a plague, with resulting devastation and a major loss of life. Aromatic woods were burned extensively on bonfires to deal with the stench of death and decay. Cloves were carried to ward off bad odours. Doctors often wore nosebags filled with cloves and cinnamon, for their protection as they tended the sick and dying.

From our more recent past, René-Maurice Gattefossé, a French chemist, discovered the antiseptic properties of aromatic oils by accident. He burnt his hand and put it into a vat of lavender oil; the wound healed quickly without blistering or scarring.[3] He wrote a book in 1928 on this subject, *Aromatherapie*.[4] A French surgeon Dr Valnet used essential oils to treat injured soldiers and calm mentally disturbed patients in psychiatric hospitals; he also wrote a book called *The Practice of Aromatherapy*.[5] The first clinic in England was established in 1950, teaching beauty therapists how to use aromatic oils for massage. Gradually aromatherapy became firmly established as an integrated and integral part of our complementary healthcare system.

Applications in modern medicine

Aromatic oil can be:

- applied to the skin as a massage treatment
- inhaled on a handkerchief or pillow or candle
- inhaled as a vapour
- added to bath water
- heated on a specifically designed oil burner
- used as a compress
- applied to skin as an oil
- ingested, such as rose hip syrup for coughs and colds.

Evidence

Aromatherapy, with its intimate touch, has been shown to have positive effect in anxiety; it has also been proven that patients treated with aromatherapy are less affected by pain and have a faster recovery rate.[1,3] Studies have also shown that aromatherapy with its many benefits has a positive effect in palliative care.[6] In addition it has shown good results in the treatment of dementia in the elderly.[7] Research has revealed its beneficial and therapeutic effects in childbirth.[8]

Common aromatic oils in use include the following:

Evening primrose oil

- To prevent dandruff
- For eczema and dry skin conditions
- To heal wounds

Tea-tree oil

- *Antimicrobial*: useful in dry scalp conditions
- *Anti-inflammatory*: to treat sinusitis, eczema, wounds, cuts, burns, aches and pains
- *Expectorant*: for coughs, colds and catarrh
- *Antifungal*: for athlete's foot, ringworm and thrush

Conditions suitable for treatment with aromatherapy

- Anxiety
- Asthma
- Depression
- Stress
- Headaches
- Hypertension
- Insomnia
- Irritable bowel syndrome
- Eczema
- Rheumatism
- Generalised stress and tension
- Musculoskeletal conditions
- Palliative care
- Childbirth

> *Wisdom is only found in truth*
>
> *Johan Wolfgang Von Goethe*

References

1 Wantraub MI (ed). *Alternative and Complementary Treatment in Neurologic Illness*. New York: Churchill Livingstone; 2001.
2 Lis-Balchin M and East H. *Aroma Science. The chemistry and bioactivity of essential oils*. Surrey: Amberwood Publishing Ltd; 1995.
3 Lis-Balchin M. Essential oils and 'aromatherapy': their modern role in healing. *J R Soc Health* 1997; 117: 324–9.
4 Gattefossé RM. *Aromatherapie. Les Huiles, Essentielles, Hormones, Vegetales*. Paris: Girardot; 1937.
5 Valnet J. *The Practice of Aromatherapy*. Saffron Walden: CW Daniel Co Ltd; 1986.
6 Dunwoody AL, Smyth A, Davidson R. Cancer patients' experiences and evaluations of aromatherapy massage in palliative care. *Int J Palliat Nurs* 2002; 8: 497–504.

7 Thorgrimsen L, Spector A, Wiles A *et al*. Aromatherapy for dementia. *The Cochrane Library Issue 3*. Oxford: Update Software; 2003.
8 Burns E, Blarney C and Lloyd AJ. Aromatherapy in childbirth: an effective approach to care. *Br J Midwifery* 2000; 10: 639–43.

Further reading

- Gould F. *Aromatherapy for Holistic Therapists*. Cheltenham: Nelson Thornes Ltd; 2003.
- Lis-Balchin M. Essential oils and 'aromatherapy': their modern role in healing. *J R Soc Health* 1997; 117: 324–9.
- Price S. *Aromatherapy Workbook*. London: Thorsons; 1993.

Contacts

- *British Association of Therapeutic Touch*: www.ttouch.org.uk; 5 Union Street, Carmarthon, Carmartonshire, Wales SA31 3DE
- *International Federation of Aromatherapists*: www.ifaroma.org; 182 Chiswick High Road, London W4 1PP

9

Ayurvedic medicine

If I have the belief that I can do it, I shall surely acquire the capacity to do it, even if I may not have it at the beginning.

Mahatma Gandhi[1]

Ayurveda, ayur, meaning life and *veda,* knowledge or science, is a traditional system of holistic medicine that is practised in India and has been widely used for around the last 6000 years. In *Ayurveda* the life force or divine energy that flows through the body maintains balance and harmony, preventing ill-health and disease. It is shrouded in mystery in the west, and perhaps because of this factor has become fashionable among the rich and famous. Aspects of *Ayurveda* have become westernised, diluted and distorted in recent years, and some of its spiritual and mystical components have become lost in order to fulfil western expectations.

History, philosophy and evidence

Ayurvedic medicine consists, in its original form, of many different components. These include diet, exercise, yoga, meditation, herbal remedies, fasting, detoxification and urine therapy. It has similar principles to traditional Chinese medicine and is just as complex, compared to our western healthcare approach.

Most Ayurvedic practitioners in the west use meditation, massage, yoga, herbs and relaxation techniques. Some include 'detoxing' methods such as strict fasting regimes and bowel-cleansing practices as part of a more western form of Ayurveda.

To try to simplify the basic principles of traditional Indian medicine, practitioners believe that the **body is made up of three main elements, known as 'doshas':**[2]

- *vata dosha*: a combination of the element of **air and space** (ether) that allows freedom of movement
- *pitta dosha*: **fire and water**, allows change or transformation. It is used for digestion and metabolism
- *kapha dosha*: this is **water and earth** and allows cohesion within structure.[2]

These elements or *'doshas'* allow all the organs of the body to work together in harmony and are used to interpret any significant imbalances. They also create a relationship with the environment, earth and universe.

A practitioner will take a detailed history and assess the state of the *'doshas'*. A thorough examination of the tongue, nails, lips, eyes, ears, mouth, genitals, rectum and heart is conducted. The seasons and the environment are also taken into account. Ayurvedic medicine is based in the physical and its earth bound elements, or *'bhutas'*, earth, water, fire and space, and seeks to restore the individual's unique constitutional balance. The *'bhutas'* have special and individual qualities. From a combination of all these elements, a person will be diagnosed according to classification, the emphasis being placed on controlling forces of the '*doshas*', which maintains balance within the body. The diagnosis is usually a combination of two elements or '*doshas*'; sometimes only one will suffice to diagnose the problem. Health is dependent on the correct balance of all three '*doshas*'. To correct any imbalance, Indian herbal remedies, yoga, meditation, diet or exercise may well be used to restore harmony to the system. Prevention of ill-health, restoring and maintaining balance is the main feature of this system of medicine – it does not cure disease. A healthy lifestyle is advocated predominantly at all times. Disharmony can occur as a result of planetary influences, stress, emotional disturbances, childhood abuse, alcohol, smoking and infection. The Ayurveda philosophy is to find out why the body has become susceptible to environmental and emotional influences creating ill-health.[2,3]

When there is disharmony, the body releases toxins that can block or restrict the flow of energy and distort the natural rhythm creating disease, hence the need for detoxification and elimination of waste from the body.

There is little research at this time on Ayurvedic herbal medicine. Care must be taken as medication is often prescribed in multiples of herbs. It is always wise to be cautious, particularly with the more vulnerable patients, in certain diseases and also to maintain an awareness of the aggressive actions of fasting and 'detox' diets on chronically ill patients (*see* 'Special awareness and precautions in Ayurdevic herbal remedies' below).

Ayurvedic medicine is used:

- to prevent ill-health
- for body detoxification
- for relaxation
- for stress relief
- to increase energy levels
- to create balance and harmony, in mind, body and spirit
- for immune system support.

> *May I become at all times, both now and forever*
> *A protector for those without protection*
> *A guide for those who have lost their way*
> *A ship for those with oceans to cross*
> *A bridge for those with rivers to cross*
> *A sanctuary for those in danger*
> *A lamp for those without light*
> *A place of refuge for those who lack shelter*
> *And a servant to all in need.*
>
> *Dalai Lama*[4]

Special awareness and precautions in Ayurvedic herbal remedies

Particular care needs to be taken in relation to:

- toxicity in general (from herbal tonics)

- pregnancy in particular, also babies, the elderly, weak and vulnerable in chronic ill-health (there should be no fasting or detoxing)
- adverse reactions and drug interactions particularly with the oral contraceptive pill, digoxin and warfarin
- bleeding disorders.

Ayurvedic herb prescriptions are usually a combination and are rarely used singly, hence the need for caution. The more commonly used single herbs in Ayurvedic medicines (*see* Table 9.1) are to be found in supermarkets and health food shops and are generally used for self-help purposes only.

Table 9.1   Single herbs used for a range of everyday common ailments

Herbs (example)	Ayurvedic name	Common uses
Cinnamon	Taj	As an appetite stimulant, respiratory problems
Myrrh	Bola	Gum disease, mouth ulcers, haemorrhoids, menstrual problems
Garlic	Lashuna	Toxin elimination, tonic, 'flu symptoms, fluid retention, stiff joints
Mustard	Rai	Backache, constipation, coughs and colds
Onions	Dungri	Colds, skin disorders, joint problems, asthma
Aloe	Kumari	Purgative, tonic, burns, inflammation
Ginger	Ardraka	Nausea, vomiting, diarrhoea, headaches, colds, influenza
Cloves	Lavanga	Colds, toothache, indigestion, asthma
Nutmeg	Jalpala	Appetite stimulant, flatulence, vomiting, stress, insomnia
Tumeric	Haldi	Immunity support, diabetes, improves circulation, anaemia

> *We cannot do great things. We can only do little things with great love.*
>
> *Mother Teresa*[5]

References

1   Gandhi D. *India Unreconciled*. New Delhi: The Hindustan Times; 1944.
2   Mishra L, Sing BB and Dagenais S. Ayurveda: a historical perspective and principles of the traditional healthcare system in India. *Altern Ther Health Med* 2001; 7: 36– 42.
3   Mishra L, Sing BB and Dagenais S. Healthcare and disease management in Ayurveda. *Altern Ther Health Med* 2001; 7: 44–50.
4   Lama D. *Ancient Wisdom, Modern World*. London: Abacus; 2000.
5   Mother Teresa. *In My Own Words*. New York: Barnes and Noble; 1997.

Further reading

- Shaw D, Leon C, Kolevs S *et al*. Traditional remedies and food supplements: a 5-year toxicological study (1991–1995). *Drug Saf* 1997; 17: 342–56.
- Dahanukar S and Thatte U. Curent status of ayurveda in phytomedicine. *Phytomedicine* 1997; 4: 359–68.

Contacts

- *Ayurvedic Medical Association UK*: 1079 Garratt Lane, Tooting Broadway, London SW17 0LN; tel: 020 8682 3876; The Golden Dome, Woodley Park, Skelmersdale WN8 6UQ; tel: 01695 51008

10

Counselling

Mindfulness ... has to do with who we are, with questioning our view of the world and our place in it, and with cultivating some appreciation for the fullness of each moment we are alive. Most of all, it has to do with being in touch.

John Kabat-Zinn[1]

Most people are aware of the uniqueness of self and their place in society. From an individual perspective we must accept ultimate responsibility for our own actions and behaviour. This is regardless of the influence of genetic make-up, society, family dynamics and the environment. Individual behaviour is the influence of personal growth and development. While everyone is affected by their circumstances, environment and family, the individual alone is held responsible for how he chooses to behave or reacts and how he lives his life.[2] Personal growth and development is the vital ingredient to understanding acceptance, compassion, integrity and awareness of self. Counselling is one of the means for the responsible individual adult to help achieve this balanced perspective.

It can never be responsible or healthy to suppress feelings and emotions particularly if they are negative. We often do not know how to express what we feel, or even recognise the feeling for what it is. Perhaps it is because of our own dysfunctional perceptions of reality, and this may well also cause a similar disconnection from our physical body. Sometimes, we can become fragmented and allow ourselves to become distracted and alienated from our inner selves. The authentic way to deal with life is through an integrated approach with the emotional lessons of the heart, a connection of mind, body and spirit. This is the key to emotional reconnection, resulting in physical and mental balance.

Counselling is about challenging the fragmented parts of the self, where we are constantly losing emotional energy and draining our vital reserves. 'Talking therapy' helps us regain control of our life without fear, anger, resentment and conflict, with renewed harmony. An empowered, emotionally connected adult does not waste energy needlessly, except in matters of compassion, love and trust.

The two most influential spokesmen on human psychology are the American psychotherapists, Carl Rogers (1902–1987) and Abraham Maslow (1908–1970). Rogers pioneered 'client-centred therapy' better known as counselling in Britain. This type of therapy allows the individual client to make his own connections without being directed, or manipulated. This in turn helps him or her develop their own personal view of the situation and to learn to handle it or, if necessary, in time change it.

Rogers thought that problems stemmed from the fact that people can get out of touch with their true selves, as a result of others whose affections and approval are conditional, such as 'You will be loved only if you please me'. Trying to live up to this type of expectation can result in a sense of failure. This scenario places a person in a position of emotional vulnerability and they become unable to admit to their true and authentic feelings. This can distort our emotional perceptions of the real world and cause long-lasting health problems. Rogerian counselling helps clients reduce their emotional dependence. They learn not to be affected by the judgement of others and in doing so help restore the value of self. Emotional intelligence refers to positive qualities like empathy, flexibility, resilience and social awareness. Success in many aspects of life from work, marriage and daily life depends very much on how we manage our emotions.

> *There appears to be a strong trend towards studying, developing and utilising*
> *these procedures which offer help in bringing to modern man an increased peace*
> *of mind. It would seem that our culture has grown less homogeneous, it gives*
> *much less support to the individual. He cannot simply rest comfortably upon the*
> *ways and traditions of his society, but finds many of the basics and conflicts of life,*
> *centering on himself. Each man must resolve within himself issues for which his*
> *society previously took full responsibility.[2]*
>
> *Carl Rogers*

Abraham Maslow had a very optimistic view of the human condition, seeing people as naturally sociable and co-operative. He believed that antisocial behaviour only occurs when people cannot fulfil their basic needs. He compiled a comprehensive list of these, starting with the most basic for our existence, *food*, *water* and *warmth*, followed by *love* and *security*, to the needs of self-development and personal growth. He decided that if these basics are met, it keeps all aspects of personality in harmony.[3]

> *The unexamined life is not worth living.*
>
> *Socrates*

Balanced adult behaviour depends on personal power and having these basic needs in place. Adults in this positive frame of mind are likely to be less defensive and are more likely to accept others, and so to be healthy is to have a high degree of personal self-acceptance and unconditional self-regard.

Unfortunately, fear often lies at the root of all dysfunction. Fear of death underlines our fear of change, simply because we cannot see what lies beyond. Counselling allows the opportunity to talk without interruption or contradiction, in confidence, without judgement or criticism, allowing the beneficial release of pent-up emotions, helping individuals to find inner peace and boost self-confidence. **To be heard and understood is the basis of emotional freedom**. It is also used to clarify situations and allows space and time to access actions of the past. This can result in the freedom to work through priorities for future reference, gaining insight to motive and needs. It can instil enough confidence to make vital decisions about life, from a more balanced and integrated perspective.

Counselling services are many and varied and found in all aspects of society, in the workplace, private clinics, schools and colleges, within the NHS in primary care and hospital settings, organisations such as Relate and in the community. There are also many voluntary organisations that offer counselling, including hospices and churches and in pastoral care.

Indicators of an existing emotional problem are that an individual has the inability to be flexible or learn from experience. It becomes a struggle to let go of the past and deal with loss from an adult perspective. There is increased difficulty in handling conflict or criticism effectively. There are generally problems with finishing projects and coping with stress. This type of individual finds it difficult to work in a team or sustain personal relationships.

Conditions suitable for therapy

- General anxiety and associated disorders. Insomnia, panic attacks, agoraphobia, phobias, social phobias, obsessive compulsive disorders
- Depressive disorders
- Post-traumatic stress disorder
- Eating disorders
- Chronic illness (coping strategies)
- Bereavement complications
- Substance abuse, alcohol, drugs
- Palliative care
- Stress
- Childhood problems, abuse
- Relationship problems
- Redundancy
- Sexual problems

Dysfunctional coping strategies presented by patients

- Anxiety, depression, hopelessness
- All things to all people all the time, 'the doormat'
- Constant approval-seeking behaviour
- Abuse or neglect of children
- Compulsive, perfectionist behaviour
- Chemical dependency, alcohol, drugs
- Suicidal tendency

The essential qualities embraced in counselling therapies[1]

- Empathy
- Unconditional positive regard
- Non-possessive warmth
- Genuineness or congruence
- Living in the here and now

To be truly whole requires harmony; it is essential to have a clear identity and know who we are and to have questioned and examined life reached up to this point in time. We need to have clear commitments, know our boundaries and limitations. Compassion and empathy for others is a must, and it is vital to show gratitude for our good fortune, for all the gifts we have and to be respectful of all living things. The regular practice of mindfulness trains us to be aware of our inner experience.

Examples of dysfunctional family rules

These situations or attitudes may lead to long-term physical and emotional health problems:[4]

- never speak freely to others about problems
- showing perfection at all times
- others come first, always
- fun, play, laughter are irresponsible
- don't do as I do, do as I say
- love is conditional
- unclear or blurred boundaries
- don't make life difficult
- everything in the 'real' world is negative.

Types of counselling

Some of the many therapeutic counselling therapies available include the following:

- counselling in primary care, generalist therapy
- cognitive–behavioural counselling therapy
- family therapy
- bereavement counselling
- relationship counselling, Relate
- group counselling/therapy
- psychotherapy, analytical therapy.

> *Words are the most powerful drug used by mankind.*
> *Rudyard Kipling, 1865–1936*

References

1 Kabat-Zinn T. *Wherever You Go There You Are*. New York: Hyperion; 1994.
2 Rogers CR. *Client Centred Therapy*. London: Redwood Books Limited; 1994.
3 Maslow AH. *Motivation and Personality*. New York: Harper and Row; 1954.
4 Stewart W. *A–Z Counselling Theory and Practice*. London: Chapman and Hall; 1995.

Further reading

- De Shazer S. *Keys to Solutions in Brief Therapy*. New York: WW Norton and Company; 1985.
- Mattick RP, Andrews G, Hadzi PD *et al.* Treatment of panic attacks and agoraphobia. An integrative review. *J Nerv Ment Dis* 1990; 178: 567–76.
- Rogers CR. *On Becoming a Person*. Boston: Houghton Mifflin; 1961.
- Subby R. *Healing the Family Within*. Florida: Health Communications Inc; 1990.
- Department of Health. *Treatment Choice in Psychological Therapies and Counselling Evidence Based Clinical Guideline*. London: Department of Health; 2001.

Contacts

- *British Association for Counselling*: 1 Regent Place, Rugby, Warwickshire CV21 2PJ
- Support and counselling services (*see* Chapter 6)

Herbal medicine

You have to see yourself at the centre of the creative process. You have to accept responsibility for all outcomes.
You have to recognise that all thoughts have consequences, even the most minor.
You have to identify with a larger self than the one living here and now in this limited physical body.

Deepak Chopra[1]

The medicinal use of herbs, plants and flowers is almost as old as mankind itself. Throughout the world it is estimated that natural herbal medicine is more commonly practised than the conventional use of modern drugs. It is estimated that around 15% of conventional medicine is plant based.[2] Herbalism in the past was thought of as fringe medicine or substitute for health care in less well-developed countries. Today there are over 1000 herbal remedies available from chemists and health food shops in the UK.[2] Many different complementary disciplines also use herbs in a variety of ways, Bach flower remedies, naturopathy, traditional Chinese medicine (*see* Chapter 20), Ayurvedic medicine (traditional Indian medicine; *see* Chapter 9) and aromatherapy (*see* Chapter 8) all depend on the medicinal properties of herbs and plants. Homeopathy and Bach remedies also use highly diluted herbs, plants and flower materials.

History and philosophy

In early civilisation, food and medicine were inextricably linked, and many herbs were consumed for their health-giving properties. Primitive tribes in many parts of the world still use traditional knowledge of plants, making use of their healing and life-sustaining properties. This information is handed down through generations. Knowledge and uses of herbs for medicinal purposes can be traced back to the ancient Egyptians, whose priests were also herbal practitioners. The slave workers of Egypt, who built the pyramids, regularly consumed garlic on a daily basis to ward off pestilence, fevers and infections on a preventive basis. A papyrus dated 1500 BC from the ancient city of Thebes lists hundreds of medicinal herbs, including cinnamon and caraway seeds which featured largely in common use and are still in evidence today.[2,3] The Roman invaders of Europe and Britain brought with them lavender and rosemary, two of the most common herbs used extensively in the art of cookery and aromatherapy.

The other major ancient cultures that relied heavily on herbs for health care were India and China. Herbal medicine in India is still very much part of their own cultural system of Ayurvedic medicine (*see* Chapter 9). The Chinese have many schools of herbal medicine and have dispensaries in most hospitals (*see* Chapter 20). It is well documented that Hippocrates the 'father of medicine' used herbs in his treatment and prevention of disease. In the west, up until the 18th century, herbs were the only form of medicine available. In medieval times in Britain, monasteries had their own herb gardens and the monks were all trained in medicinal herbalism and treated both the monks and the local communities. Palaeontologists have discovered many herb seeds and flower fossils at ancient sites, evidence suggesting that herbs and plant life were essential for human existence.[2]

We must continue to gather knowledge and skills in the use of medicinal plants and herbs for modern society and for sustaining life in the future. There is a danger that we may over-harvest nature's bounty, resulting in a depletion of the earth's life-giving plants. These therefore must be used wisely, and the more information that is available generally, the safer the consumer will be in their use, particularly in self-medication. The side-effects are significantly less than from conventional drugs, but nevertheless vigilance is necessary when using any form of herbal medication. The safest approach to herbal medication is through qualified medical herbalists who are up to date on drug and other interactions.

Medical herbs can be used as analgesics, relaxants, anti-inflammatory agents, antidepressants, antibacterials, and as support for the immune system. Most of the medicinal herbs are used for prevention, to help boost the immune system.[4] Herbs, as with all medicines, have a placebo effect. We are all affected to some degree by advertising in the media and glossy magazines to follow the latest health trends, to hold back the ravages of time and look younger and feel better. This fuels the need for a tonic or mood enhancer and a potion or lotion to sustain this modern trend.

Herbal remedies are many and varied, taken internally or applied externally. The most common preparation is the infusion, which is prepared from fresh or dried leaves where flowers and stems are soaked in boiling water and used to make herbal tea. Many preparations are in tablet and capsule form made from dried herbs. Capsules need less processing of the materials used to make them. Tinctures are a common form and are highly concentrated and used over a period of time, for example a few drops in a glass of water perhaps on a daily basis. This and herbal tea consumption is considered the safest way to take herbal medicine, as the amount taken is diluted. Herbs can also be used externally as a soothing bath or applied locally as a cream, ointment, compress or poultice, which can be applied to any part of the body and used extensively in essential oils for aromatherapy.

It is estimated that in the UK alone we spend £126 million on herbal remedies annually. The World Health Organization (WHO) has stated that the world market for herbal medicines is worth £41 billion.[5] This is staggering in monetary terms, but equally worrying is our herbal avarice and the rate of depletion and exploitation of the more exotic and rare plant materials used from around the world.

Application in modern medicine

Most of the herbs for the conditions below can be bought in supermarkets and health food shops, for example, Aloe vera for irritable bowel syndrome, St John's wort for anxiety and depression. Agnus castus is used for treating symptoms of menopause. The following conditions are all suitable for self-help medication:

- anxiety/depression
- acne

- abrasions
- arthritis
- athlete's foot
- catarrh
- colds, coughs
- cramps
- cystitis
- dandruff, alopecia, dry scalp
- diarrhoea
- dyspepsia, reflux, indigestion
  insomnia
- eczema, dry skin
- flatulence
- fungal infections
- haemorrhoids
- halitosis
- influenza, fever
- irritable bowel syndrome
- menopause
- morning sickness
- mouth ulcers
- pain
- premenstrual syndrome and menstrual problems
- prostate problems
- rheumatism
- sinus problems
- stress
- sunburn
- thrush
- tooth and gum disorders
- urticaria, heat rash, pruritus
- worms.

Case study 11.1: Feverfew

Jane is a 59-year-old lady with a 20-year history of debilitating migraines, which generally lasted for at least 2 to 3 days out of every month. She was confined to bed in a darkened room. Jane could never predict when or what would trigger her migraines and had already tried all the conventional drugs available. Some had worked for a short time but none gave her the freedom to make too many long-term plans. She was given Feverfew tablets to take when she developed an attack, or at the onset of the prodromal signs. She had significant relief from Feverfew, but it did not stop the number of attacks. Homeopathic Natrum muriaticum as a prevention remedy was then given every three to six months and this worked well. For the last year Jane's migraines are under control with this combination of the herb Feverfew and Natrum muriaticum, a homeopathic remedy.

Evidence: some of the medicinal herbs validated by clinical trials

Black cohosh (Cimcifuja racemosa)

This is a very well-known female remedy. It is also used homeopathically as Actea racemosa or Black snakeroot (tincture of the root) for depression during the menopause and also in intercostal myalgia. Black cohosh is a very prominent herb sold as a complementary remedy to alleviate menopausal symptoms.

Most clinical trials were done in Germany. In a multicentre study, 629 women with menopausal symptoms, each received 40 drops of Black cohosh twice daily for 6–8 weeks. There was an 80% improvement at 4 weeks. Good tolerance was reported by 93%, with no side-effects.[6–8]

Vitex agnus castus

This is an extract from the fruit of Vitex agnus castus (VAC) of the Vitex chaste tree or chasterbury. It has long been used to help with symptoms of premenstrual, menstrual and menopausal symptoms. A multicentre non-interventional trial (open study without control) was carried out to test the efficacy and tolerance of Agnus castus under routine medical conditions, and the study used 1634 patients who had symptoms of premenstrual syndrome (PMS). After three menstrual cycles, 93% of sufferers reported a decrease in the number of symptoms or even cessation of PMS symptoms. This result was observed in all symptom complexes. There were no serious drug adverse reactions, hence the risk/benefit ratio of the Vitex agnus castus was noted as significant efficacy in all aspects of the multifaceted and homogenous clinical picture of PMS.[9]

A further study using leaf and fruit of Agnus castus for menopausal balance was carried out on 23 participants; the results were very positive in the relief of common menopausal symptoms.[10]

Garlic (Allium sativa)

Most people are familiar with the garlic bulb, particularly in the flavouring of food, where it is usually used in a similar way to onions. It has a long history around the world as a 'cure all' and it is true to say garlic has been used to treat a great number of ailments. Garlic is rich in Alliin and other sulphur compounds, and has been shown to have an anticoagulant effect and to lower cholesterol.[11] Research has also shown positive effects on infections.[12,13] Clinical studies confirm garlic's efficacy on bacteria, viruses, fungi and worms, if it is taken over a long period of time.[13]

Aloe vera

The name Aloe vera stems from the Arabic word *alloeh*. There are more than 500 species of this plant and four types with known medicinal properties. The plant, which is considered most potent and is the one most referred to in scientific circles, is Aloe barbadensis milla also known as Aloe vulgaris or Curacao aloe. Around 75 chemical compounds are found in the plant, including minerals, amino acids, sugars and enzymes.[14] Aloe vera has also a proven anti-inflammatory effect.[15] Studies show Aloe has emollient moisturising and antimicrobial properties.[16]

Feverfew

An ancient herb that grows wild and in many gardens in the UK has been used in the past for fevers, arthritis and migraine.[17] It is in migraine and headaches where Feverfew has been found to be of most value.[18] It is not fully understood exactly how it works but research suggests that sufferers with low level of circulatory melatonin may be more prone to migraine attacks. Feverfew is thought to boost levels of melatonin.[18,19]

Saw palmetto

This is a dwarf palm tree native to the West Indies and United States and is used mainly in the treatment of benign prostatic hyperplasia (BPH). It is thought to work by the same mechanism as conventional drugs, by blocking the production of the enzyme 5-alpha reductase used to change testosterone into dihydrotestosterone (DHT).[20–22]

Echinacea

This is mostly used to treat coryza, influenza, herpes and catarrh. It is widely used to boost the immune system. The root extract of Echinacea has been shown to have interferon-like activity and antiviral properties.[23–25] Studies have shown that Echinacea can help to relieve symptoms and reduce the severity of coryza. Researchers are divided as to whether it is useful in the prevention of coryza.

St John's wort (Hypericum perforatum)

This has been used extensively in mild to moderate depression, anxiety and in seasonal affect disorder (SAD). The herb works in part by increasing serotonin, and is therefore not used with conventional antidepressants such as selective serotonin re-uptake inhibitors (SSRIs).[26,27] Studies have revealed that St John's wort should not be used in pregnancy,[26–28] and it has also been reported to produce photosensitivity in some individuals.

Ginkgo biloba

Clinical trials have shown that standardised Ginkgo biloba extracts (GBE) have significant uses in the treatment of increased intestinal permeability, senile dementia, depression, tinnitus, glaucoma, cataracts, vascular insufficiency and macular degeneration. It is thought to act on and improve the circulation generally, and has an anticoagulant effect.[29,30] Clinical trials on the treatment of dementia have been promising, particularly in memory impairment and lack of concentration.[30]

Love Creates Healing.

Sanaya Roman[31]

References

1   Chopra D. *How to Know God*. New York: Rider; 2001.
2   Capasso L. 5300 years ago, the Ice Man used natural laxatives and antibiotics. *Lancet* 1998; 352: 1864.
3   Vickers A, Zolman C. ABC of complementary medicine. *BMJ* 1998; 319: 1050–3.
4   Craig WJ. Health promoting properties of common herbs. *Am J Nutr* 1999; 70: 4915–95.
5   World Health Organization. *WHO Traditional Medicine Strategy 2002–2005*. Geneva: World Health Organization; 2002. www.who.int/medicines/publications (accessed 11 October 2006).
6   Dukar E, Kopanski L, Jakry H *et al*. Effects of extracts from Cimcifuja Racemosa on gonadotropin release in menopausal women and ovariectomized rats. *Planta Med* 1991; 57: 420–4.
7   Cottlieb B. *New Choices in Natural Healing*. Emmaus PA: Rodale Press Inc; 1995.
8   Vonberg G. Treatment of menopause symptoms. *ZFA* 1984; 60: 626.
9   Loch FG, Selle H and Boolity NJ. Women's health. *Gend Based Med* 2000; 3: 315–20.
10 Chopin Lucks B. Vitex agnus castus essential oil and menopausal balance: a research update. *Complement Ther Nurs Midwifery* 2003; 8: 148–54.
11 Berthold HK, Sudhop T and von Bergman K. Effect of a garlic oil preparation on serum lipoproteins and cholesterol metabolism: a randomized controlled trial. *JAMA* 1998; 279; 1900–2.
12 Adetumbi M and Lau B. Allium sativum (garlic): a natural antibiotic. *Med Hypoth* 1983; 12(3): 227–37.
13 Tynecka Z and Gos Z. The inhibitory action of garlic (Allium sativum L) on growth and respiration of some micro-organisms. *Acta Microbiol Pol B* 1973; 5: 51–62.
14 Lorenzetti LJ, Salisbury R, Beal JL *et al*. Bacteriostatic property of aloe vera, *J Pharm Sci* 1964; 53: 1287.
15 Udupa SL, Udupa AL and Kulkarni DR. Anti-inflammatory and wound healing properties of aloe vera. *Fitoterapia* 1994; 65: 141–5.
16 Davis RH, Leitner MG, Russo JM *et al*. Aloe Vera a natural approach for treating wounds, oedema and in diabetes. *J Am Podiatr Med Assoc* 1988; 78: 60–8.
17 Murch SJ, Simmons CB and Saxena PK. Melatonin in feverfew and other medicinal plants. *Lancet* 1997; 350: 1598–9.
18 Murphy JJ, Heptinstall S and Mitchell JR. Randomized double-blind placebo-controlled trial of feverfew in migraine prevention. *Lancet* 1988; 2: 189–92.
19 Johnson ES Kadam NP, Hylands DM *et al*. Efficacy of feverfew as prophylactic treatment of migraine. *BMJ* 1985; 291: 569–73.
20 Carraro JC, Raynaud JP, Koch G *et al*. Comparison of phytotherapy (Permixon) with finasteride in the treatment of benign prostatic hyperplasia: a randomised international study of 1098 patients. *Prostate* 1996; 29: 231–40.
21 Albrecht J and Sokeland J. A combination of sabal and urtica extracts vs finasteride in BPH (stage 1 to 11 Acc to Alken): a comparison of therapeutic efficacy in a one-year double-blind study. *Urologe* 1997; 36: 327–33.
22 Overmyer M. Saw palmetto shown to shrink prostatic epithelium. *Urology Times* 1999; 27: 42.
23 Hoffman D. *The New Holistic Herbal*. Shaftsbury: Element; 1990.
24 Melchart D, Walther E, Linde K *et al*. Echinacea root extract for the prevention of upper respiratory tract infections; a double-blind placebo controlled randomised trial. *Arch Fam Med* 1998; 7: 541–5.
25 Grimm W and Muller HH. A randomized controlled trial of the effect of fluid extract of Echinacea purpurea on the incidence and severity of colds and respiratory infections. *Am J Med* 1999; 106: 138–43.
26 De Smet PAGM and Nolen WA. St John's Wort as an anti depressant. *BMJ* 1996; 313: 241–2.
27 Linde K, Ramirez G, Mulrow CD *et al*. St John's Wort for depression – an overview and meta-analysis of randomized clinical trials. *BMJ* 1996; 313: 253–8.
28 Wheatley D. L1 160, an extract of St John's Wort, versus amitriptyline in mild to moderately depressed outpatients – a controlled 6-week clinical trial. *Pharmacopsychiatry* 1997; 30(suppl): 77–80.
29 Kleijnen J and Knipschild P. Gingko Biloba. *Lancet* 1992; 340: 1136–9.

30 Hopfenmuller W. Proof of the therapeutical effectiveness of Ginkgo biloba Special extract: Meta-analysis of 11 clinical trials in aged patients with cerebral insufficiency. *Arzneim Forsch* 1994; 44: 1005–13.

31 Roman S. *Spiritual Growth. Being Your Higher Self.* California: HJ Kramer Inc; 1989.

Further reading

- British Herbal Medicine Association. *A Guide to Traditional Herbal Medicine: a source book of accepted traditional uses of medical plants within Europe.* Bournemouth: British Herbal Medicine Association; 2003.
- Mills S and Bone K. *Principles and Practices of Phytotherapy: modern herbal medicine.* Edinburgh: Churchill Livingstone; 2000.
- Mills S and Bone K. *The Essential Guide to Herbal Safety.* Edinburgh: Churchill Livingstone; 2005.

Contacts

- *British Herbal Medicine Association*: www.bhma-info; Field House, Lye Hole Lane, Redhill, Bristol BS18 7TB
- *International Register of Consultant Herbalists*: 32 King Edward Road, Swansea SA1 4LL; tel: 01792 655886
- *Medicines and Healthcare products Regulatory Agency (MHRA)*: www.mhra.gov.uk
- *National Institute of Medical Herbalists*: www.nimh.org.uk; 56 Longbrook Street, Exeter, Devon EX4 6AH
- *National Institute of Medicinal Herbalists*: Elm House, 54 Mary Arches Street, Exeter EX4 3BA; tel: 01392 426022

12

Homeopathy

> *To know men is to be wise, to know oneself is to be illuminated. To conquer men is to have strength, to conquer oneself is to be stronger still. And to know when you have enough is to be rich.*
>
> *David Baird*[1]

The healing art

Homeopathy is derived from the Greek (*homeo* meaning similar and *pathos* meaning disease). Hippocrates first thought of and documented the idea of using Cantharis (Cantharis vesicatoria) to treat 'strangury' (cystitis), thus establishing the basic homeopathic principle of 'treating like with like'. This describes the law of similars, a fundamental principle of homeopathy. In Latin the phrase *'similia similibus curentur'* translates 'let like, cure like'.

Dr Samuel Hahnemann, a Leipzig physician born in the 18th century, developed the idea further and established homeopathy in Germany and eventually world-wide.

> *There are no diseases only sick people.*
>
> *Samuel Hahnemann (1755–1843)*[2]

Hippocrates and Hahnemann, therefore, observed long ago the importance of the holistic approach. The individual presenting with symptoms is, first and foremost, more important than the disease itself.

Homeopathic remedies are used in treating both acute and chronic diseases. There are many benefits in using homeopathy in primary and secondary care. It is a form of therapeutics, whereby the properties of plants, poisons, minerals, metals and extracts from diseased tissue are harnessed and used safely for the benefit of mankind.

Homeopathic remedies

When homeopathic remedies are produced, the original substance, a plant for example, is pounded and made into a concentrated 'mother tincture'. From there, the substance is diluted and succussed (a 'shaking' process) serially until the substance is so dilute that no molecules are present in the diluent (Avogadro's law in molecular biology). However, the active physical 'memory' is thought to be imparted to the diluent in the succussion process. This is the method thought to help remedies gain their activity. The more dilute the remedy, the more potent it becomes as it is subjected to this succussion and dilution process. This is why there are low- and high-potency homeopathic remedies.

Homeopathic remedies have no side-effects or toxicity on the body. Remedies are safe to use in all age groups, including pregnant women.

As of September 2006, the Medicines and Healthcare products Regulatory Agency (MHRA) implemented a new regulation allowing the inclusion of therapeutic indications for over-the-counter (OTC) homeopathic medicines.

Mode of action

The theory of how homeopathic remedies are active is different from that for orthodox medical treatments. Conventional medicine suppresses infections with antibiotics, pain with analgesics and emotions with anxiolytics. Homeopathic remedies stimulate the immune system and the healing abilities of the body into resolving infections, pain, emotional problems and so forth. Healing therefore takes place by 'natural' means by harnessing the body's own powers. The balance is therefore restored to the normal healthy state.[3]

A homeopathic physician (homeopath) will take a conventional medical history in detail and also record the homeopathic history, examine the patient, investigate appropriately and arrive at a diagnosis. During the homeopathic assessment, the homeopath will gather details of what is known as the symptom complex. This is the recognition of a collection of symptoms, which are then matched as closely as possible to a homeopathic remedy.

This matching of the symptom complex to the patient's symptoms is done manually using the *Materia Medica* or by computer, and is known as repertoirising. Usually there are a number of matches, and the remedy that is nearest to the match is selected for treating the patient.[4]

Steroids, coffee, mints and homeopathy

Steroids, mint and coffee all block the action of homeopathic remedies. Patients are advised to reduce or stop taking coffee and to use a non-mint-containing toothpaste when taking remedies. If a patient is taking steroids and is unable to discontinue them, then a homeopath will prescribe a higher potency remedy for a longer period of time.

Homeopathic treatment

The holistic approach in treating a patient with homeopathy can best be illustrated in the management of a child with scarlet fever.[5]

The symptom complex of a child presenting with scarlet fever is that of an ill-looking febrile child, with a flushed skin, displaying circum-oral pallor and derma-tographia. The tongue is coated, and the pharynx may have follicles on the tonsils. There is lethargy, the pupils are wide, and despite a high fever there is no thirst and the child is chilly and wanting to be wrapped up. A homeopath will note all these symptoms and make the diagnosis of scarlet fever, and in addition note (from the symptom complex) that this is a case for Belladonna (deadly nightshade). Giving a homeopathic preparation of Belladonna will often cure the patient. Giving the same remedy to other members of the family may actually prevent the onset of scarlet fever. Homeopathy, therefore, has not only a therapeutic role but also a preventive one.

How does Belladonna cure the patient?

The remedy is thought to act on the body's immune defence system to produce a cure. The remedy acts as a 'trigger' to restore the individual to health in the same way that the disease acts as a 'trigger' to tip the balance into scarlet fever.

Why is Belladonna chosen for this particular disease?

It is known from toxicology that Belladonna is a poisonous plant, and when it is ingested in significant amounts the very same symptom complex as scarlet fever occurs. In the last century children died of scarlet fever before attenuation of the streptococcal strain occurred, which reduced the disease to a milder form to the extent that it is now often called 'scarletina'. If a diluted homeopathic preparation of Belladonna is used to treat a patient, there are no side-effects and the properties of the remedy are harnessed to produce a cure. Other diseases producing a similar symptom complex of fever and flushing, as in sunburn, scalds and viral infections (such as fifth disease) can also be helped by Belladonna.

The remedies are administered sublingually at frequent intervals for acute conditions. When the patient improves clinically and the infection is deemed resolved, the remedy is stopped. Homeopathic remedies are cost-effective,[6] are available on an FP10 prescription form, and any chemist can obtain them from one of the homeopathic manufacturers.

The conventional treatment for scarlet fever is penicillin, the antibiotic of choice, and paracetamol as an antipyretic. Both drugs rely on gastric absorption and adequate blood levels to achieve an impact on the *Streptococcus* bacterium causing the infection. Often in the febrile child, conventional drugs can induce vomiting, necessitating the intramuscular route for administering the antibiotic and leading to hospital admission. A 5–7-day course of antibiotics is normally prescribed in this instance. This can be contrasted with a course lasting a few hours to a few days of a sublingually administered single homeopathic remedy that is palatable and has no toxic effect.

Treating pain

In the treatment of pain, homeopathy takes account of the *modalities* as well as the *type* of pain, for example in joint problems, if the pain is 'better for movement' Rhus toxicodendron (Poison ivy) is used. If the pain becomes worse on movement, Bryonia (Wild hops) is prescribed. For 'tearing' pain in a ligament Ruta gravis (Garden rue) is indicated. In sciatica, Hypericum (St John's wort) relieves the pain. It is therefore, crucial that an accurate and detailed homeopathic history is taken to match the remedy to the symptoms.[7–9]

Treating psychological problems

In the treatment of emotional problems, homeopathy is very beneficial. There is no sedation or other side-effects but, as with all treatments in homeopathy, there may be 'an aggravation' where some symptoms may 'surface', becoming worse before they get better. This aggravation could apply to physical symptoms, such as joint pains, as well as emotional problems. An aggravation can last a few hours to a few days before improvement takes place.

In the sections on anxiety (*see* Chapter 2), depression (*see* Chapter 4) and bereavement (*see* Chapter 6) examples are given where homeopathy can be used. Instead of *suppressing* feelings by the use of anxiolytics, homeopathy seeks to *release* emotions such as anger, resentment and tearfulness, thus calming and eventually *healing* the whole person.

Chronic disease

It is in the treatment of chronic disease that homeopathy has potential to alleviate and cure in many patients.[10] The homeopathic history produces the symptom complex, which is then matched to the individual patient in choosing the remedy and the potency.[11] Psychological, social and environmental factors are also taken into account.

Obviously no system of medicine can claim to cure all diseases, but even incurable disease symptoms can be alleviated by skilful use of homeopathic remedies (*see* Chapter 29). Counselling and lifestyle changes are just as important in homeopathy as they are in conventional medicine.

Constitutional remedies

Homeopaths recognise many more 'constitutional profiles' than the conventional division between type A and type B personality groups. These constitutional remedies often need to be used in the treatment of chronic illness.

Argentum nitricum, Chamomilla, Lachesis, Lycopodium, Natrum muriaticum, Nux vomica, Phosphorus, Pulsatilla, Sepia, Staphysagria, Sulphur and Thuja described in this chapter are some examples of constitutional remedies. The symptom complex of each of these remedies can be matched to recognised patterns of personality types.

The symptom complex

To help understand this, a selection of remedies is described in order to appreciate the diversity and detail of the symptoms in homeopathic history taking to enable a remedy match to be made. Each remedy will be described as a symptom complex (cluster of symptoms), showing the homeopathic use in various medical conditions. This is known as *Materia Medica*, the known properties of a remedy, which can be matched to the patient's symptom complex to arrive at a homeopathic prescription.

The homeopathic remedy guide

The *Materia Medica* is a compilation of homeopathic remedies, which can be equated with the pattern of the patient's symptoms.[4] This uses the 'like with like' principle to select the correct remedy for a patient.

Only a small selection of remedies is included here for demonstration purposes. A brief outline of each remedy is given to enable the reader to gain an understanding of how homeopathic prescribing takes place. There are around 200 commonly prescribed remedies and over 2000 listed.

Usually a low-potency remedy is used for an acute or localised condition and a higher potency for a chronic physical or emotional problem. The choice of remedy depends on the person's personality type and the homeopathic details obtained in the history taking and observations made during the examination of the patient.

The six most important symptoms are repertoirised (remedy matched) to identify the remedy or remedies that closest match in the 'like with like' principle. The one with the highest score is usually chosen for the patient. Each symptom (called a rubric) is ranked in order of importance. Repertoirising can also be done by computer, which selects a list of matched remedies.[4]

Arnica montana (Leopard's bane)

The patient feels bruised all over and may have contusion, stiffness and muscular pain. Symptoms are made worse by the slightest touch. The main use is in trauma, postoperatively, during childbirth and soft tissue injuries. This is a useful remedy for excessive fatigue following exercise.

Aconite napellis (Monkshood)

This is commonly used in anxiety, fright, shock and sensitivity to touch and restlessness that is out of proportion to the situation. In an acute illness with fever, at the onset of an infection, a few doses of Aconite napellis can be given, followed by other remedies indicated as the infection progresses.

Argentum nitricum (silver nitrate)

Patients in this symptom complex are usually thin, have difficulty remembering things, and are constantly excited, in a hurry and worried. They feel time passes too quickly and want to get everything over with, due to lack of confidence. There is usually anticipatory anxiety and also a craving for sweet food. Vertigo in high places is also a common symptom.

Arsenicum album (white oxide of arsenic)

This is useful in pale, thin cold-sensitive individuals, who display weakness, restlessness and worry. They have a great need for heat. Individuals who would benefit from Arsenicum are fastidious, in other words orderly to the point of obsession, and alternate between excitement, depression and mood swings. They sometimes have generalised burning pains. Usually symptoms are worse (this is known as an *aggravation* in homeopathic terms) in the early hours of the morning, typically 1–3 am. Thirst for frequent small amounts of cold water is a common feature. Nervous restlessness can be accompanied by fear of death for no apparent reason. Arsenicum is indicated in presentations of influenza where the patient is pale, very cold with loose stools and rhinorrhoea, asthma, gastroenteritis, eczema, psoriasis, anxiety and depression.

Cantharis (Spanish fly)

This is a common remedy used for cystitis with frequency and dysuria. Cantharis is also indicated in haemorrhagic cystitis, burns, scalds and erysipelas. A midstream specimen of urine should be analysed to ensure complete resolution of the infection, as would occur in conventional medical management.

Chamomilla

This is used for hyperaesthesia and sensitivity to pain out of proportion to the seriousness of the condition. The patient is irritable, easily angered, moody and often with a very disagreeable nature. It is indicated in nervous adults, who cannot tolerate anyone or anything and who are hypersensitive to pain. In a child, the condition often improves by being carried or when travelling in a car. It is often used for symptoms of teething and otitis media.

Hypericum (St John's wort)

This is the remedy for nerve ending pain, therefore is used widely in neuritis, sciatica and also postoperatively. It can be helpful in post zoster neuralgia and depression. It is useful for postoperative pain and is usually given with Arnica.

Ignatia (St Ignatius bean)

In this symptom complex there is hypersensitivity with fainting, moodiness or sudden outbreak of anger. Sadness, tearfulness, ruminating and deep sighing are often present. The remedy is indicated at the initial stages of grief and for the onset of globus hystericus.

Ipecac (Ipecacuanha root)

This is used in respiratory and gastrointestinal infections especially for spasmodic coughs resulting in nausea and vomiting and the exacerbation of asthma with wheezing. Nausea in pregnancy can also be controlled with this remedy.

Lachesis (Bushmaster snake)

The Lachesis type of patient often has left-sided symptoms such as headaches/ migraine. The patient can be loquacious with a jealous streak and a tendency to bleed easily. In PMS this remedy can alleviate the symptoms of fluid retention (bloating of the abdomen and mastodynia). Often the woman is unable to bear tight clothing around the neck, has difficulty getting off to sleep and dreams of snakes, death and funerals. The cyclical symptoms usually improve with the onset of menstrual flow. It is used to treat hot flushes at the onset of menopause. Mild to moderate essential hypertension can also be treated with this remedy.

Lycopodium (Club moss)

Patients are intellectually keen but sometimes physically 'weak'. Symptoms are aggravated (made worse) between the hours of 4 and 8 pm. It is indicated in dyspepsia, duodenal ulcer, flatulence, bloated abdomen and chronic urticaria. Symptoms are predominantly right sided. There is often a craving for sugar, sweets and a preference for warm drinks. The person is often warm to the touch. There is a sudden lack of confidence and mental irritability after a 'cat nap'. This is one of the main remedies used in anticipatory anxiety and irritable bowel syndrome.

Mag phos (magnesium phosphate)

This is used when pains begin and end suddenly and are cramp-like or neuralgic in nature. Spasmodic and sharp at times the patient doubles up to get relief from pain. The symptoms are predominantly right sided. It is indicated in dysmenorrhoea, sciatica, facial neuralgia, writer's cramp and colicky-type pains in general.

Natrum muriatiacum (sea salt)

Typically, this remedy is used where there is grief, disappointed love, depression and introversion. Often the patient complains of weakness and weariness, a dry mouth causing thirst, and a preference for savoury food. Consolation causes an aggravation with weepiness. There is a fear of being rejected or hurt emotionally.

Headaches, cold sores, geographical tongue, PMS and menopausal symptoms also respond well to this remedy.

Nux vomica (Poison nut)

This is used in individuals who are very irritable, impatient, hypersensitive, have sleep disturbances (waking around 3–4 am), and are chilly and want to be covered to keep warm.

It is indicated in stress due to overwork, hangovers, dyspepsia, spasmodic back pain and constipation.

Phosphorus (The element)

A 'phosphorus patient' is indifferent, full of fears and anxiety, does not like to be alone or in the dark, is fidgety and alternates between excitement and depression. They experience burning sensations, crave salt, cold food and drinks. A cough can be elicited going from warm to cold air. Usually talkative, they are deathly afraid of storms, and symptoms are worse at dusk. Phosphorus is used in anxiety, depression, asthma, laryngitis, viral hepatitis and alcoholic polyneuritis. It is indicated in haemorrhages following dental extractions and epistaxes in children.

Pulsatilla (Pasque flower)

A patient who will respond to Pulsatilla as a constitutional remedy is usually female, blonde, blue eyed and fair skinned. Menarche is often later than usual. This person never hurries, is easy-going, resigned, moody, shy and gentle in nature. They display feelings of sadness and a tendency to cry. Symptoms are generally worse in heat and they cannot tolerate the hot sun, which often results in a headache. They are better for being outside in fresh air and moving about. A Pulsatilla-type personality is not generally thirsty, they like and feel better for consolation. This remedy is very useful for chilblains, catarrh, dysmenorrhoea, coryza, otitis media, dyspepsia and flatulence with bloating. It can also be used in PMS and in menopausal symptoms.

Sepia (Cuttlefish ink)

Although this is used mostly in females it can help males who fall into the Sepia constitution. It is described as the 'washerwoman's' remedy. She can be pale, sweating, tired and depressed, with a marked indifference to loved ones, self-neglect and a reduction in libido. She displays marked tiredness, making everything a great effort, with menstrual disorders and a bearing-down feeling in the pelvis. There is a sensation of emptiness present in the stomach. This is one of the main remedies used in the menopause and PMS.[12] Sepia is one of a number of remedies used to treat headaches.[13]

Staphysagria (Stavesacre)

This is indicated in bottled up anger, repressed indignation, humiliation or sadness. The patient is very sensitive to the slightest word, excitable and easily irritated. The patient never becomes angry however and is therefore nervous. There are burning pains in the urethra with frequency of micturition. Staphysagria is useful in honeymoon cystitis, chalazion and lacerated wounds. In patients who are resentful, this remedy helps calm this emotional state, restoring a peaceful mind.

Sulphur

Sulphur constitutions are very warm (bodily), philosophical in outlook, have large appetites and like to eat the fat on meat. They have a tendency to constipation. The patient is often anxious, untidy and sluggish in nature, they are usually worse for heat, and wilt in the sun. Sulphur is indicated for symptoms that are hot or burning. This is a remedy often used in chronic illness such as asthma and eczema, and also the menopause for hot flushes.

Thuja occidentalis (Arbor vitae)

This remedy constitution is likened to the 'Narcissistic syndrome'.

In a significant reaction following immunisation, Thuja can relieve the symptoms.

In the treatment of warts with Thuja, the result can be quite dramatic. Chronic anxiety, catarrh, sinus infections and polyps can also be treated with this remedy.

In modern medicine, emphasis has evolved away from individual patients, concentrating more on diseases and their management. For research purposes this is important, but it is often at the expense of the patient. Through homeopathy it is possible to tailor treatments to the individual. It is this individualisation of symptom complexes that make double-blind placebo-controlled trials so difficult in the study of homeopathy (*see* Chapter 32). Nevertheless, outcome studies are reported to enable a scientific evaluation to be made, showing that remedies have been proven to be effective (*see* Chapter 32).

Homeopathy is therefore a system of therapeutics that makes use of naturally available organic and inorganic materials. Over the decades, science has removed much of the art of medicine and there is a danger of tipping the balance more and more towards bigger and better technology and forgetting the most basic human needs of communication, understanding and empathy in the healing process.[14]

References

1   Baird D. *A Thousand Paths to Wisdom*. London: MQ Publications Ltd; 2000.
2   Hahnemann S. *Organon of Medicine*. London: Victor Gollancz Ltd; 1986.
3   Chapman EH. Homeopathy. In: Weintraub MI (ed). *Alternative and Complementary Treatment in Neurological Illness*. Philadelphia: Churchill Livingstone; 2001.
4   Kent JL. *Repertory of Homeopathic Materia Medica and a Word Index*. London: Homeopathic Book Service; 1986.
5   Demetriou A. Homeopathy in practice In: Gray DJP (ed). *The Royal College of General Practitioners Members' Reference Book*. London: Sterling Publications Ltd; 1990. pp. 415–16.
6   Jain A. Does homeopathy reduce the cost of conventional drug prescribing? A study of comparative prescribing costs in general practice. *Br Homeopath J* 2003; 92: 71–6.
7   Van Haselen RA and Fisher PAG. A randomised controlled trial comparing topical piroxicam gel with a homeopathic gel in osteoporosis of the knee. *Rheumatology* 2000; 39: 714–19.
8   Zell J, Connert WD, Mau J *et al*. Treatment of acute sprains of the ankle joint. Double-blind study assessing the effectiveness of a homeopathic ointment preparation. *Fortschr Med* 1988; 106: 96–100.
9   Bell IR, Lewis DA, Brooks AJ et al. Improved clinical status in fibromyalgia patients treated with individualized homeopathic remedies versus placebo. *Rheumatology* 2004; 43: 577–82.
10 Spence DS, Thompson EA and Barron SJ. Homeopathic treatment for chronic disease: a 6-year, university-hospital outpatient observational study. *J Altern Complement Med* 2005; 11: 793–8.
11 Murphy R. *Homeopathic Remedy Guide* (2e). Virginia: HANA Press; 2000.
12 Yakir M, Kreitler S, Brzezinski A *et al*. Effects of homeopathic treatment in women with premenstrual syndrome: a pilot study. *Br Homeopath J* 2001; 90: 148–53.
13 Muscari-Tomaioli G, Allegri F, Miali E *et al*. Observational study of quality of life in patients with headache, receiving homeopathic treatment. *Br Homeopath J* 2001; 90: 189–97.
14 Dixon M, Sweeney K. *The Human Effect in Medicine*. Oxford: Radcliffe Publishing; 2000.

Further reading

- Boyd H. *Introduction to Homeopathic Medicine*. Beaconsfield: Beaconsfield Publishers Ltd; 1981.
- Chapman EH, Weintraub RJ, Milburn MA *et al*. Homeopathic treatment of mild traumatic brain injury: a randomised, double-blind, placebo-controlled clinical trial. *J Head Trauma Rehabil* 1999; 14: 521–42.
- Gerhard I and Wallis E. Individualized homeopathic therapy for male infertility. *Homeopathy* 2002; 91: 133–44.
- Papp R, Schuback G, Beck E *et al*. Oscillococcinum in patients with influenza-like syndromes: a placebo-controlled double-blind evaluation. *Br Homeopath J* 1998; 87: 69–76.
- Reilly D, Taylor MA, Beattie NGM *et al*. Is evidence for homeopathy reproducible? *Lancet* 1994; 344: 1601–6.
- Reilly D. The evidence for homeopathy. Glasgow Homeopathic Hospital, January 2003. www.adhom.com

- Tveiten D, Bruseth S, Borchgrevink CF *et al*. Effects of the homeopathic remedy Arnica D30 on marathon runners: a randomized double-blind study during the 1995 Oslo Marathon. *Complement Ther Med* 1998; 6: 71–4.
- Tyler ML. *Homeopathic Drug Pictures* (3e). Essex: Daniel CW; 1952.
- Weatherley-Jones E, Nicholl JP, Thomas KJ *et al*. A randomised controlled, triple-blind trial of the efficacy of homeopathic treatment for chronic fatigue syndrome. *J Psychosom Res* 2004; 56: 189–97.
- White A, Slade P, Hunt C *et al*. Individualised homeopathy as an adjunct in the treatment of childhood asthma: a randomised placebo controlled trial. *Thorax* 2003; 58: 317–21.
- Weiser M, Strosser W and Klein P. Homeopathic vs conventional treatment of vertigo: a randomised double-blind controlled clinical study. *Arch Otolaryngol Head Neck Surg* 1998; 124: 879–85.

Contacts

- *British Homeopathic Association*: www.trusthomeopathy.org; Faculty of Homeopathy, Hahnemann House, 29 Park Street, Luton LU1 3BE
- *Royal London Homeopathic Hospital*: Greenwell Street, London W1W 5BP
- *The Society of Homeopaths*: www.homeopathy-soh.org; 11 Brookfield, Duncan Close, Moulton Park, Northampton, NN3 6WL

13

Hypnotherapy

By learning to contact, listen to, and act on our intuition, we can directly connect
to the higher power of the universe and allow it to become our guiding force.
Shakti Gawain[1]

The name hypnosis comes from the Greek *hypnos,* meaning sleep. The definition of
hypnosis is the induction of a state in which a person's normal critical or sceptical
nature is bypassed, allowing the acceptance of suggestions. It is a state of mind that
can occur naturally through daydreaming (while awake), or is established by compliance with instruction.

Hypnosis appears to encompass altered states of consciousness, such as daydreaming, meditation or intense concentration. Meditation is self-directed and may
qualify as hypnosis, depending on the state achieved. Daydreaming is authentic and
can be a regular pre-occupation, where the mind state is altered to a different
frequency and engaged in personal fantasies and at the same time awake and
aware, but oblivious to the external world of movement and its many distractions.
Hypnosis can therefore occur naturally without formal induction.

Hypnosis, as a technique, allows the state of altered consciousness, a daydream
state, to be achieved formally, and directs the attention to focus on specific goals in
order to achieve them. Like daydreaming, hypnosis is a perfectly normal, safe and
healthy approach to problem solving. Such hypnotic or 'trance'-like states are
characterised by an increased receptivity to verbal and non-verbal communications, which are usually referred to as 'suggestions'.

Hypnosis helps to:

- focus attention
- heighten receptivity
- bypass the sceptical nature of the mind
- receive acceptable suggestions
- create balance between conscious and subconscious
- deliver acceptable suggestion

and can also be used as an investigative tool.

History and philosophy

The history of hypnosis in the west started in France in 1778. An Austrian physician
Franz Anton Mesmer used 'animal magnetism', the original term used for mes-
merism or present-day hypnosis. He believed that by using magnets it was possible
to improve and restore good health, cure illness and balance the body. As time
progressed, he became discredited as a performer and showman and for giving
medicine a disreputable name. Just as in today's society where there are numerous

stage performances and shows where hypnosis is used to sabotage human integrity, this behaviour does not in any way discredit the therapeutic range and effectiveness.

James Braid, using eye fixation techniques, produced a trance-like state. He subsequently refined this process of hypnosis and added suggestion. Today he is credited with the name of hypnotism.[2,3]

In the 19th century the English surgeon John Elliotson and a Scottish surgeon James Esdale performed hundreds of surgical procedures using hypnosis instead of conventional anaesthesia. This resulted in a very low morbidity for that period of time.[4] Eventually ether and chloroform displaced the use of hypnosis in surgery.[5] In 1955 the British Dental and Medical Hypnosis Society was established.

In 1958 the American Medical Association (AMA), reported from a study that lasted for two years conducted by the Council of Mental Health, stated that there should be 'definite and proper use of Hypnosis in Medical and Dental practice'. The AMA recommended the establishment of 'necessary training facilities' in the United States.[6,7]

The British Medical Association (BMA) had issued its own report on hypnosis in the *British Medical Journal*, agreeing with the AMA's findings.[8] In 1991 the American Psychiatric Association stated that 'hypnosis has definite application in the various fields of medicine' and that physicians would be interested in finding psychiatrists to train in hypnosis.[8]

A German neuropsychiatrist Hans Berger (1873–1941) demonstrated by electroencephalography (EEG) that when the eyes are closed the brain generates regular waves (measured in cycles per second) (cps). These were called *alpha* waves and subsequent discoveries resulted in the identification of *theta, beta* and *delta* waves, also found in various mental functions and activities. Experts disagree on basic numbers of cps for different wave formations. It is commonly regarded that the range between 0 and 4 cps is total unconsciousness. Little is known about this level. *Theta* ranges between 4 and 7 cps. It is thought that all our emotional experiences are recorded in *theta* and that this level is beyond hypnosis and leading into the world of psychic experiences. *Alpha* falls between 7 and 14 cps, and is regarded as the subconscious range, where dreaming (while asleep) and nearly all hypnosis takes place, meditation is also achieved mostly at this level. *Beta* is the frequency of the conscious mind (14 cps) and upwards. This is generally the awake and physically functional stage – making decisions, being active – and operates at about 20 cps during active periods. It is thought that around 60 cps would be in the realm of hysteria. Hypnosis can induce the brain to move into *alpha* without a state of sleep, where the subconscious mind is open to suggestions so does not reason or think, and is in a perfect state for hypnosis.[9,10] The theory of hypnosis is not yet fully understood nor is it understood exactly how the subconscious mind follows instructions.

In a hypnotic state, tasks are performed effectively and efficiently. Instructions are obeyed, vocal communication is constructed and lucid. Therapists can use this to help bring about physical or emotional changes in a client's health. Hypnosis can be used to induce relaxation, reduce pain, or gain an insight into problems and past events, which may well help resolve present difficulties. It is fairly common for a client to be taught self-hypnosis following resolution of an illness, for example asthma or irritable bowel syndrome, to use as a backup in the prevention of a recurrence. For positive outcomes and for hypnosis to work well, it is essential that the patients actually want to be hypnotised of their own free will.

People with chronic pain can actually lose the memory of the pre-pain state; it becomes part of their daily existence and their personality. It is believed that hypnosis can regress the mind to a time when the mind and body were pain-free, to enable the patient to re-experience these lost feelings. Hypnotherapy can provide suggestions that help create new patterns for living and set free the presenting physical and mental symptoms. The common therapeutic uses of hypnosis at present are for pain relief, relaxation and addiction. It is particularly popular for nicotine withdrawal. It is also widely used as a regression technique as part of psychotherapy, providing a key to unlocking emotional blocks through repressed memory. Hypnosis has recently become popular in past life regression therapy as a means of resolving present problems.

Applications in modern medicine

Hypnosis is used for the following:

- asthma
- musculoskeletal conditions
- anxiety
- amnesia
- sleep disorders
- sexual dysfunction
- phobias
- addictions
- depression
- stress
- palliative care
- childbirth
- postoperative surgery for pain relief
- essential hypertension
- irritable bowel syndrome
- psychotherapeutic regression
- post-traumatic stress syndrome.

Evidence

There have been numerous studies in the use of hypnotherapy for pain relief, with positive results and with significant relief, especially for burn injuries in children.[11] Also, patients with recalcitrant temporomandibular joint pain treated with hypnosis in jaw relaxation noted significant pain reduction.[10,12] Hypnosis in childbirth, used as anaesthesia, has a long successful history, with many positive trials reporting less discomfort and shortened labour.[13]

An oral surgeon documented his own cholecystectomy using self-hypnosis only for his anaesthetic; he walked back to his room following surgery and subsequently returned to work on the 10th postoperative day.[14]

There are very encouraging studies in gastroenterology. Hypnosis is used particularly in irritable bowel syndrome to improve patients' quality of life, and investigators have reported a significant reduction in absenteeism from work following hypnosis.[15,16]

Hypnosis is used to combat nausea and other adverse effects, particularly following chemotherapy. Results showed less nausea but also a reduction in anticipatory nausea, and decreased vomiting.[17] According to a recent study, hypnosis is useful in the care of the elderly with phobic problems, reducing the need for medication.[18]

> *Look back on your life,*
> *Now look ahead in your life*
> *Now look inside your life.*

Author unknown

References

1   Gawain S. *Living in the Light*. New York: Bantam; 1993.
2   Spiegel H, Greenleaf M and Spiegal D. Hypnosis. In: Sadock BJ, Sadock VA, *Kaplan & Sadock's Comprehensive Textbook of Psychiatry*. Volume 2 (7e). Philadelphia: Lippincott Williams and Wilkins; 2005. pp. 2138–46.
3   Forest DW. *Hypnotism: a history*. London: Penguin; 1999.
4   Marmer MJ. Present applications of hypnosis in anaesthesiology. *West J Surg Obstet Gynecol* 1961; 69: 260–3.
5   Blankfield RP. Suggestion, relaxation and hypnosis as adjuncts in the care of surgery patients: a review of the literature. *Am J Clin Hypn* 1991; 33: 172–86,
6   Scientific status of refreshing recollection by the use of hypnosis. Council of Scientific Affairs. *JAMA* 1985; 253: 1918–23.
7   Durbin PG. *Kissing Frogs: practical uses of hypnotherapy* (2e). Dubuque, Iowa: Kendall/Hunt Publishing Co; 1998.
8   American Psychiatric Association. *Regarding Hypnosis* position statement (approved by the council, 15 February 1961). www.psych.org/public_info/libr_publ/position.CFM (accessed 11 October 2006).
9   Gidro-Frank L and Bowersbuch MK. A study of plantar response in hypnosis regression. *J Nerv Ment Dis* 1948; 107: 443–58.
10 LeCron LM. A study of age regression under hypnosis. In: LeCron LM (ed). *Experimental Hypnosis: a symposium of articles on research by many of the worlds' leading authorities*. New York, NY: Macmillan; 1952. pp. 155–74.
11 LaBaw WL. Adjunctive trance therapy with severely burned children. *J Child Psychother* 1973; 2: 80–92.
12 Simon EP and Lewis DM. Medical hypnosis for temporomandibular disorders: treatment efficiency and medical utilization outcome. *Oral Surg Oral Med Oral Pathol Oral Radiol Endod* 2000; 90: 54–63.
13 Jenkins MW and Pritchard MH. Hypnosis: Practical applications and theoretical considerations in normal labour. *Br J Obstet Gynaecol* 1993; 100: 221–6.
14 Rausch V. Cholecystectomy with self-hypnosis. *Am J Clin Hypn* 1980; 22: 124–9.
15 Whorwell PJ, Prior A and Faragher EB. Controlled trial of hypnotherapy in the treatment of severe refractory irritable bowel syndrome. *Lancet* 1984; 2: 1232–4.
16 Houghton LA, Heyman DJ and Whorwell PJ. Symptomatology, quality of life and economic features of irritable bowel syndrome: the effect of hypnotherapy. *Aliment Pharmacol Ther* 1996; 10: 91–5.
17 Zeltzer LK, Dolgin MJ, Le Baron S *et al*. A randomised, controlled study of behavioural intervention for chemotherapy distress in children with cancer. *Pediatrics* 1991; 88: 34–42.
18 McIntosh I. Hypnosis: a useful tool in the medical care of older people. *Geriatr Medicine* 2006; 36: 17–20.

Contacts

- *British Society of Medical and Dental Hypnosis*: www.bsmdh.org; 17 Keppel View Road, Kimberworth, Rotherham, South Yorkshire S61 2AR; tel: 07000 560 309
- *The Hypnotherapy Association*: www.thehypnotherapyassociation.co.uk
- *The National Council for Hypnotherapy*: www.hypnotherapists.org.uk
- *National School of Hypnosis and Psychotherapists*: Central Register of Advanced Hypnotherapists, 28 Finsbury Park Road, London N4 2JX; tel: 020 7359 6691

14

Massage

To contain our energy is to embrace our bodily excitement, to let feelings unfold within our containing body and to let ourselves be formed by these feelings. By living with and from our bodily feelings, they change us, altering our love.
Stanley Keleman[1]

The healing power of the hands has been known and used for centuries. Massage is one of a number of hands-on healing techniques used in modern day medical care. It is gradually becoming recognised for its therapeutic value and is now more widely used, to extend the hand of human compassion in a healing context. Touching is a very physical activity, we do it instinctively and it has hidden therapeutic affect of which we are not always aware. It is a form of natural communication of feelings with a partner, children, family and friends. Massage is an extension of this innate human ability that can also be interpreted as having a huge emotional significance. If we have a pain or ache, we automatically rub or massage the area to soothe and relieve the pain. For example, in headaches we use our hands to massage the neck and temples instinctively; it is almost a reflex action. The same with a child, a parent or carer will instinctively rub and stroke the painful area, the pain will often subside leaving the child feeling better than before, because of the added injection of love and attention.

The mind and body work together; physical ailments such as headaches are quite often a reflection of what is in the mind. Muscles release and tighten in response to emotional difficulties such as anger, frustration, anxiety, fear, grief; the body then relaxes when the emotional problem is dealt with and resolved. The physical body acts like a receptacle for a lifetime's emotions and experiences including birth, childhood trauma, illness, pain, shock and loss. This includes all that has happened to our emotional and physical body from birth until death.

We cannot heal what we cannot feel.
John Bradshaw[2]

It is not enough for the psyche to acknowledge sadness or anger, emotional release must fully involve the body's whole structure and mechanisms. There is movement associated with each emotion, and until the movement is freed up, the energy of the emotion will remain in the physical body. We use touch in daily life during normal contact with family and friends. It is used as a comforter for people who are suffering from stress, anxiety or depression, and in times of loss and grief. Touch is essential for growth and development from birth to adulthood. A mother touches, holds and comforts as a means of passing on love, security and comfort; from this a child will feel secure and accepted, and will thrive, grow and develop.

History and philosophy

The history of massage from ancient records has been attributed to being one of the oldest forms of physical medicine known to man. Present knowledge is unclear as to where the word originates. It is thought that the Arab word *mash* means to press softly, or the Greek word *massein*, 'to knead', or the French *masseur*, translates to 'shampoo'. There is also evidence that the Greek and Roman physicians, Socrates, Plato and Heroditus used massage extensively in their work. Hippocrates, 'the father of medicine', wrote that 'rubbing can bind a joint that is too loose and loosen a joint that is too rigid, hard rubbing binds, much rubbing causes parts to waste and moderate rubbing makes them grow'. Pliny, a Roman naturalist, was massaged regularly to alleviate his asthma. Julius Caesar suffered from headaches and neuralgia – apparently he used massage on a daily basis. Massage and its therapeutic uses as a form of medicine have a long and varied history.

A Swedish professor Henriks Ling (1776–1839) developed a technique known as 'Swedish massage'. It was introduced to America by Dr Mitchell around 1877 and was extremely popular in medical circles. In 1894 the Society of Trained Masseurs was established in Great Britain, but, unfortunately, by 1934 this society became the Chartered Society of Physiotherapists. At this stage therapeutic massage was more or less replaced by physiotherapy.

Massage today is firmly established both in sports injury and in therapeutic touch in holistic care. At the present time it is largely practised by professional masseurs in private clinics, health clubs, hospices and hospitals as an integral part of physical therapy and general health care. Masseurs have a rigorous training and are health professionals in their own right.

Evidence

Massage has a positive effect on patients with nausea who are undergoing chemotherapy.[1] It also helps relieve anxiety in palliative care and has proven effectiveness in relieving chronic low back pain.[3–6] Studies on therapeutic touch have shown it has positive effects on infants whose mothers have postnatal depression.[5] Research has shown the benefits of therapeutic touch on irritable bowel syndrome and demonstrated the many benefits of therapeutic touch in terminal cancer care.[7,8]

Shiatsu

Shiatsu means 'finger pressure', originated in Japan and is a form of massage and pressure point therapy. Based on a combination of massage techniques, Chinese meridian theory and western anatomy and physiology, it focuses on the use of the fingers and palms of the hand to apply pressure to particular sections on the surface of the body. This is for the purposes of correcting imbalances and for maintaining and promoting good health. It is also a method of contributing to the healing of specific illnesses. In 1940 the first school of Shiatsu was established in Tokyo, and by 1953 it was introduced to the USA by Dr B Palmer, father of chiropractic medicine.

Table 14.1   Medical application of massage

System	Use
Reproductive	Abdominal and back massage to help: PMS, menopause, dysmenorrhoea and pregnancy
Genito-urinary	Helps to stimulate kidney activity to: eliminate waste products, reduce fluid retention
Digestive	Helps eliminate waste products from the bowel, prevents constipation Helps absorption where the digestion is sluggish
Respiratory	Slows and calms the breathing, promoting relaxation Helps expel secretions from the lungs in chronic chest problems
Muscular	Relaxes and contracts muscles, relieving tension Reduces muscle cramp and fatigue Used for breakdown of muscle adhesion and scars Extensively used in sport in prevention of muscle strain and injury
Skeletal	Increases blood and lymph supply to the bones Benefits nutrition and growth of bone Reduces stiffness of joints and increases flexibility
Lymphatic	Eliminates waste products Reduces oedema by disposing of waste to lymph glands
Circulatory	Helps increase circulation Reduces blood pressure Strengthens heartbeat
Nervous	A soothing and sedative effect in anxiety and fear Stimulating effects on a depressed system, reducing lethargy and fatigue
Skin	Sweat and sebaceous glands are stimulated, to improve the function of skin Encourages the skin to 'breathe' more freely Increases skin tone and texture Improves suppleness and elasticity increasing flexibility Enhances the 'feel good factor'

Applications in modern medicine

- Anxiety and insomnia
- Neuralgias
- Rheumatoid arthritis
- Muscular atrophy, paralysis, joint deformity
- Stress reduction and health promotion
- Dislocations and sprains
- Chronic constipation

Massage is commonly used for:

- pain relief, relaxation, palliative and cancer care
- headaches, particularly those that are stress related (cranial head massage is quite popular)
- muscular or joint problems, stroke recovery, cerebral palsy
- an aid to relaxation
- sports injuries: for relief and prevention

- stress related problems, irritable bowel syndrome, insomnia, chronic fatigue syndrome
- depression
- chronic anxiety
- pain relief during childbirth
- newborn babies whose mothers have postnatal depression
- in mothers with postnatal depression
- bereavement.

Contraindications

- Communicable diseases, tuberculosis (TB), gonorrhoea, syphilis
- Heart disease
- Acute illness with fever
- Cancers, sarcomas

> *Your Body speaks its Mind.*
>
> *Stanley Keleman*[9]

Reference

1 Keleman S. *Love: A Somatic View*. Berkeley, CA: Center Press; 1994.
2 Bradshaw J. *Bradshaw on the Family: A Revolutionary Way of Self-Discovery*. Deerfield Beach: Health Communications Inc; 1988.
3 Brown PR. *The Effects of Therapeutic Touch on Chemotherapy – Induced Nausea and Vomiting*. Nevada: University of Nevada; 1981.
4 Kemp L. *The Effects of Therapeutic Touch on the Anxiety Levels of Patients with Cancer Receiving Palliative Care*. Canada: Dalhousie University; 1994.
5 Glover V. Benefits of infant massage for women with post-natal depression. In: Darnell P, Pinder M and Treacey K (eds). *Searching for Evidence: complementary therapies research*. London: The Prince of Wales Foundation for Integrated Health; 2006. pp. 27–8.
6 Prayde M. Effectiveness of massage therapy for sub-acute low back pain: A randomised controlled trial. *CMAJ* 2000; 162: 1815–20.
7 Cooper RE. *The Effect of TT on Irritable Bowel Syndrome*. New York: Clarkson College; 1977.
8 Giasson M and Bouchard L. Effects of therapeutic touch on the well being of persons with terminal cancer. *J Holist Nurs* 1998; 16: 383–98.
9 Keleman S. *Your Body Speaks its Mind*. Berkeley, CA: Center Press; 1975

Further reading

- Jonas WB and Crawford J (eds). *Healing Intension and Energy Medicine*. London: Churchill Livingstone; 2003.
- Montague A. *Touching: the Human Significance of Skin*. New York: Harper and Row; 1971.
- *The Complementary Health Care: a guide for patients*. London: The Prince of Wales Foundation for Integrated Health; 2005. www.fih.org.uk (accessed 12 October 2006).

Contacts

- *General Council for Massage Therapy (GCMT)*: www.gcmt.org.uk; Whiteway House, Blundells Lane, Rainhill, Prescot L35 6NB; tel: 0151 430 8199; email: gcmt@btconnect.com

- *Sports Massage Association*: www.sportsmassageassociation.org; PO Box 4437, London SW19 1WD; tel: 020 8545 0851; fax: 020 8404 8261; email: info@thesma.org

15

Meditation

Our deepest fear is not that we are inadequate, our deepest fear is that we are powerful beyond measure. It is our light, not our darkness, that most frightens us. We ask ourselves 'who am I to be brilliant, gorgeous, talented, fabulous?' Actually who are you not to be? You are a child of God. Your playing small doesn't save the world. There is nothing enlightened about shrinking so that other people won't feel insecure around you. We are all meant to shine, as children do. We were born to make manifest the glory of God that is within us. It is not just some of us; it's in everyone. And as we let our light shine, we unconsciously give other people permission to do the same. As we are liberated from our fear, our presence automatically liberates others.
   Nelson Mandela, in his inaugural speech as President of South Africa, 1994

In India and Asia, meditation has been practised for centuries. The Buddhist way of life is based on meditation and it is used as a tool for enlightenment. Since the 1960s, meditation, like yoga, has become more commonplace in the west. It still has connotations of mysticism and we need to continue to dispel the belief that you have to be a Buddhist to meditate. It is now used regularly, the world over, by Christians, Jews, Muslims and Buddhists in the belief that we cannot make ourselves happy by improving our external world; only by finding inner peace do we truly thrive.

Meditation is highly regarded by many regular practitioners. It is used as a supreme self-help method of harnessing energy, power and mind control, using no more than our own abilities to concentrate, focus and control our thoughts and emotions to calm and slow the body. The mind has the ultimate power of control; to balance emotions we have to cultivate awareness so we can respond appropriately. Being at the mercy of moods can leave us extremely vulnerable with fewer choices. With inner balance we can handle any situation that may arise, appropriately. Physical relaxation is essential to meditation. Tension and relaxation are in fact responses of the central nervous system. It is the fight or flight response that switches on the rush of adrenaline and cortisol giving us enough energy to face the crisis in hand. Relaxation is the process that turns 'off' the stress hormone, which is the total reverse, and turns 'on' the 'relaxation response'. This mechanism is controlled by the mind at all times, depending on need. The stress response speeds up and relaxation slows down, so energy is being used up under stress and conserved during relaxation. To be effective, meditation has to be practised regularly for long-term health benefits, but can be very valuable in the shorter term in learning and gaining degrees of control. Sogyal Rinpoche, a Tibetan Lama, makes the analogy of the mind 'To a jar of muddy water, the more we leave the water without interfering or stirring it, the more particles of dirt will sink to the bottom, letting the natural clarity of the water shine through'.[1]

Regular meditation alleviates symptoms in the following:

- headaches
- anxiety, panic attacks
- chronic disease and palliative care
- insomnia
- raised blood pressure: it can help control mild essential hypertension
- stress symptoms, such as irritable bowel syndrome
- asthma, particularly in breath control
- depression: it helps improves concentration
- coronary heart disease: it is useful in prevention and management.

Benefits of meditation in ill-health prevention

- Creates mental balance.
- Can bring beauty and wisdom.
- Helps connect the mind and body, to gain control.
- Creates peace and calm.
- Focuses attention.

If you can breathe, you can meditate. It is free, can be practised alone or in a group and has no known side-effects. Under one's own control, it is easy to do and can be practised almost anywhere. There are a number of meditation techniques including focusing on the breath, repetitive sound, Mantra and visual imaging.

> *Blessed are they that have not seen and yet have believed.*
>
> *John 20:29*

Physiology of meditation

Breathing changes dramatically when we relax. When we have tense feelings, we overbreathe from the upper chest. As we relax fully, breathing usually becomes lighter and the muscles start to soften and sag as the adrenaline rush fades. This is often more apparent in the face and shoulders, then the rest of body starts to feel heavy. The circulation improves and there is an increase in blood flow to the skin, which can feel warm. The adrenaline and endorphins that are produced when there is tension of mind and body then recede when in a relaxed state. Sometimes at this stage, aches and pains are more readily felt, as they were previously masked by endorphins.

The following is an example of a simple 5 or 10 minutes' meditation. **If you can sit, don't stand, if you can lie, don't sit.**

- Sit or lie in a comfortable position.
- Close your eyes and take deep breaths, allow your breathing to be slow and relaxed.
- Focus all your attention on breathing and take note of the movement of your chest and abdomen in and out.
- Block out feelings, thoughts and sensations. If your attention wanders, remember your breathing again.

- As you breathe in, say the word 'calm' (to yourself), as you breathe out, say the word 'peace'.
- As you become relaxed, draw out the pronunciation of the words so that it lasts for the whole breath the word 'calm' 'c-a-l-m-m'. As you breathe the word 'peace' 'p-e-e-e-a-a-c-c-e'. Repeat this for the duration of the meditation.
- Always return the focus to the breath.

This is a very simple example of how easy it is to learn to focus on breathing through meditation; you can concentrate on objects such as a candle flame, a flower, a photograph or a holy icon. Joining a meditation group can take it to a deeper level with many more benefits, while at the same time reducing the isolation factor.

Meditation is about choosing where you direct your attention, shutting out all other thought processes, learning to calm the mind and body in order to relax. In doing so, we gain much more self-control. **We will become stronger in the knowledge of our own self-belief, which will lessen the need to control everything and everyone in order for our needs to be met.**

The purpose of this chapter is to simplify and de-mystify this art form of mind control in order to promote its value in health promotion. As breath is essential for life it is extremely important to learn how to use it for our own personal advantage. The simple message here is 'if you can draw breath you can meditate'.

Evidence

Regarding clinical efficacy, it was reported that the effects of meditation promote 'detached observation' and an uncoupling of the sensory dimension of the pain experience from the affective/evaluative alarm reaction.[2] The result of the many studies on the positive effect of meditation is the association with the reduction in serum cortisol, catecholamines and the positive effect in palliative care.[3,4]

Meditation has also been proven to have a positive effect in the prevention of coronary heart disease.[5]

> When we cannot see our way out of the forest, we may need to climb to the top of the mountain.
>
> Anodea Judith[6]

References

1 Rinpoche S. *The Tibetan Book of Living and Dying*. San Francisco: HarperCollins; 1992.
2 Kabit-Zinn J. An outpatient program in behavioural medicine for chronic pain patients based on the practice of mindfulness meditation: theoretical considerations and preliminary results. *Gen Hosp Psychiatry* 1982; 4: 33–47.
3 Galois P. Hormonal changes during relaxation. *Encephale* 1984; 10: 79–82.
4 Van Tilburg E. Meditation and palliative care. *CHAC Rev* 1991; 19: 9–12.
5 Ormish D, Scherwitz LW, Billings JH *et al*. Can lifestyle changes reverse coronary heart disease? The Lifestyle Heart Trial. *Lancet* 1990; 336: 129–33.
6 Judith A. *Eastern Body, Western Mind*. Berkeley, CA: Celestial Arts; 1996.

Further reading

- Farrow JT, Herbert R. Breath suspension during the transcendental meditation technique. *Psychosom Med* 1982; 44: 133–53.
- Gyatso KG. *The New Meditation Handbook* (4e). Ulverston: Tharpa Publications; 2003.
- Harrison E. *The 5 Minute Meditation*. London: Piatkus; 2003.
- Hittleman R. *Guide to Yoga Meditation*. New York: Bantam Books; 1981.
- Kabit Zinn J. *Wherever You Go. There You Are*. New York: Hyperion; 1994.

Contacts

- *Friends of the Western Buddhist Order of London*: www.fwbo.org; Buddhist Centre, 51 Roman Road, London, E2 0HU; tel: 0845 458 4716
- *Transcendental Meditation UK*: tel: 08705 41 3733; www.t-m.org.uk

16

Osteopathy and chiropractic: physical manipulation therapies

In the development of this character structure, the muscular system of the growing child is subverted from its natural function of movement to the neurotic function of holding.

Alexander Lowen[1]

Osteopathy is one of the physical manipulation therapies and has been used as a 'hands-on' musculoskeletal method of healing since ancient times. The basic principle is that the smooth and unrestricted movement of the musculoskeletal system is the key to fitness and positive good health. It was part of Eastern and European medical traditions. Both osteopathy and chiropractic emerged in the late 1800s and early 1900s in America.

The body's largest system is its framework of bones, joints, muscles and ligaments, which plays a major role in physical movement and activity. Osteopathy aims to diagnose and treat the mechanical problems of the framework. The theory is that when the structure of the body is sound and balanced, it should work like a finely tuned engine, with the minimum of wear and tear. Osteopaths believe that the musculoskeletal system is important because it is related to the autonomic nervous system, connecting all the muscles, tendons and organs throughout the active body. The function of all these depends on the free flow of nerve impulses, energy and blood supply. The parasympathetic nervous system is responsible for maintaining the rhythmic and dynamic balance of the body.

The constant upright position of the physical body automatically creates a great strain on the overall mechanism of the whole mechanical structure. Also, the force of gravity, bad posture and general wear and tear creates imbalances for the spinal vertebrae, which have to become weight bearing in the upright position. This also puts strain on the supporting discs and surrounding structures, giving rise to mechanical and physical health problems.

History and evidence

Doctor Andrew T Still (1828–1917) devised a system of manipulation techniques. This became known as osteopathy from the Greek words *osteo* meaning 'bone' and *pathos*, disease. The aim is to rebalance the framework of the body, improve joint mobility and help the functions of the internal organs. This is based on the structure of the body and its functions, which are closely connected. A spinal imbalance or restricted movement causes pain and discomfort and also interferes with the function of the internal organs. Correction of the imbalance and improving the range of movements can, therefore, ease and improve organ function.

Dr Still was an engineer as well as an army surgeon; his three children died of meningitis, which led him to devise a less physically aggressive technique for preventing disease and maintaining good health. Dr Still was fully convinced that the body was a self-regulating, self-healing organism. He was the first to realise the dynamic structure of the body in relation to its function. In his view it was the fact that the joints were properly aligned with the spine that played a vital role in supporting the whole structure of the body. The Greeks and Romans were also aware of the role of the spine in maintaining good health. Many practitioners of Chinese medicine and Indian Ayurveda also acknowledged the benefits of gentle manipulation of joints and tissues. Dr William Sutherland (1873–1954) refined Still's ideas and is credited with proving that even the bony skull is in a constant dynamic state of motion, and that the tissues, organs and bones have a unique rhythm of ebb and flow and are continuously expanding and contracting in a harmonious state. Osteopathy was originally thought of in terms of a neck and back therapy, and is viewed as a mechanical cure for cause and effect of musculoskeletal problems only. Today's osteopaths believe that soft tissue manipulation can improve energy flow throughout the body. Some of the most popular techniques widely used at present are the Bowen technique, cranial osteopathy and chiropractic.

The role of the osteopath and chiropractic is to treat and diagnose problems with ligaments, muscles, joints and nerves, recognising that much of the pain and disability stems from an abnormality of the body's structure. About 50% of patients who visit an osteopath are treated for back problems. If acute conditions are treated earlier, chronic problems can be avoided. Osteopathy can relieve pain and distress and reduce drug dependency, minimising the cost of treatment for side-effects. Osteopathic treatment does not involve the use drugs or surgery. This therapy is designed to ease pain, reduce swelling and improve mobility. Early intervention negates the necessity for further medical input.[2]

Evidence for the use of manipulation techniques

Studies have shown the positive outcomes for manipulation therapies. Spinal pain is the most common and is frequently disabling. A randomised controlled trial was carried out in primary care in a group of practices in North Wales: 201 patients with neck and back pain of 2–12 weeks' duration were studied. Tested against the usual GP care for back pain, one group received osteopathy in a health centre setting. Two months later, the osteopathy group had more improvements than the usual care group. The study concluded that in a primary care osteopathy clinic, treatment improved short-term physical and long-term psychological outcomes.[3]

A recent trial in the US and the UK, based at the Osteopathic Research Centre, collated evidence used in six trials involving eight osteopathic manipulation therapies (OMT) versus control treatment. The comparisons included blinded assessment of low back pain in ambulatory settings. It concluded that OMT significantly reduces low back pain. The level of pain reduction was greater than expected, regardless of whether trials were performed in the UK or US, and showed significant pain relief in the short and intermediate term, and at long-term follow-up.[4] A controlled trial of cervical manipulation for migraine was conducted in New Zealand. Volunteers suffering from migraine were randomly allocated spinal manipulation by a chiropractic or mobilisation by a medical practitioner or physiotherapist. The chiropractic group reported much less pain associated with their migraine attacks.[5] Children have been shown to benefit from manipulative therapies. A research trial of 316 infants found that chiropractic treatment improved symptoms of colic in 94% of the babies observed.[6]

Conditions that can be treated with osteopathy

- Arthritis
- Asthma
- Musculoskeletal conditions: spine, hips, neck, sciatica, dislocations
- Balancing and realigning of the whole system
- Tennis elbow
- Pain relief in general, especially low back pain
- Migraines

The Bowen technique

The Bowen technique was developed in Australia. It is a much more gentle form of hands-on-type of osteopathic healing. This is a muscle- and connective-tissue based energy healing. Dr Tim Bowen was an industrial chemist who became an osteopath and developed the Bowen technique. It is a specific form of massage, carried out by moving the thumbs and fingers across various tendons and muscles. This is an extremely delicate manipulation, forming a rolling action, creating energy throughout the body, and blocking and stopping the energy at various points. The deliberate creation of pauses gives the tissues time to deal with the energy created. This technique is often used in low back pain and the treatment of frozen shoulder syndrome.[3,7]

The Alexander technique

This is a method of retraining the body's movements and positions in order to improve or correct bad posture. It is used to relieve headaches, back and neck pain and relieve stress. The technique was devised by Frederick M Alexander (1869–1955), who was an actor and, through his own experiences of losing his voice on stage, believed that if you learned to improve your posture your body will work in a more natural, relaxed and efficient manner. It is widely used today by musicians, dancers, athletes and actors.

Chiropractic

History and philosophy

Chiro: Greek meaning hand; *practic*: practical.

This form of manipulation therapy places more emphasis than osteopathy on the spine, and therapists use X-ray and other diagnostic tools. Daniel Palmer (1845–

1913), founder of the Palmer School of Chiropractic, believed that 'displacement of any part of the skeletal frame may press against nerves which block the channels of communication, intensifying or decreasing their energy capacity, creating either too much or not enough functioning, an aberration known as disease'. The main aim of chiropractic is to correct joint and muscle disorder, particularly of the spine, which can induce referred pain to other parts of the body, for example the shoulder, arms, legs, and hips.

John McTimoney (1914–1980) devised a more gentle, whole-body manipulation technique using very delicate touch to correct the alignment of bones and joints to restore nerve function, alleviate pain and promote better physical body health. McTimoney practitioners firmly believe that chiropractic techniques can even be used on neonates.

Conditions suitable for chiropractic therapy

- Tension headaches
- Frozen shoulders
- Joint sprains
- Sports injuries
- Tennis elbow
- Knee injuries
- Arthritis
- Asthma
- Deafness/dizziness
- Damaged ligaments

Cranial osteopathy

This form of manipulation has many similarities with the laying on of hands and other touch techniques. The therapist combines healing with anatomical knowledge, using the hands to feel or 'listen' for restrictions and strains or stresses in the physical body. Cranial osteopathy, by virtue of the name, implies head massage and manipulation. The technique can also be used to treat the whole body. Dr Sutherland devised the system for correcting restrictions of the cranial bones using manipulation. He studied this concept by carrying out his theories and experimenting on himself. Dr Sutherland kept detailed records of all the symptoms, which included depression and head and jaw pain that were a direct result of the head restriction he created himself. The original focus was on the bones of the skull, and in time it became apparent that other body parts were involved, particularly the sacrum. If the pelvis is tilted, twisted or unbalanced in any way, it will have a direct effect on the sacrum and its attachments, including the spine and base of the cranium.

The cranio-sacral approach evolved from cranial osteopathy and includes awareness of the effects of emotional stress on the body. During this gentle therapy, an osteopath senses and manipulates using 'energy' in a manner that is in many ways similar to that of other forms of energy healing. This technique is safe to use on babies and young children, who often respond well to treatment.

Osteopathy in infants and children

Common problems in infants

- Feeding problems
- Sickness, colic and wind
- Sleep disturbances
- Crying and irritability

Common problems in children

- Musculoskeletal conditions
- Susceptibility to infections, low immune system
- Chronic ear infections, glue ear
- Sinus and dental problems
- Migraines/headaches, aches and pains
- Asthma, chest conditions
- Behavioural problems, learning difficulties, poor concentration, hyperactivity
- Cerebral palsy, Down's syndrome

Statistics for back pain in the UK (The UK Osteopathic Information Service)[7]

- It is the UK's leading cause of disability.
- Four out of five people suffer back pain, lasting more than a day, at some point in their lives.
- Back pain is common in **children**. Around 50% of children in Europe experience back pain at some time.
- It is estimated that £480 million each year is spent on services used by sufferers of back pain, which includes 14 million consultations, seven million therapy sessions and 800 000 hospital beds.
- Back problems and repetitive strain injury cost British industry £5 billion annually.
- Doctors issue around 55 million prescriptions for analgesics and non-steroidal anti-inflammatory drugs annually.

Prevention of back problems

- Regular physical activity in the form of regular exercise.
- Avoid being overweight to reduce strain on the musculoskeletal frame.
- Avoid repetitive tasks, vary rhythm and take regular breaks.
- Pace and be realistic about heavy physical work and activity.
- Avoid strain when lifting: there is a right/wrong way to lift safely.
- On long car journeys, take regular breaks to move about and stretch.
- Change the mattress at regular intervals to suit the back, avoiding potential problems.
- In pregnancy correct posture and rest is important.

- Many hours spent in one position will result in long-term problems, such as leaning over a desk, or working on computers.

> *There is a chorus that says, 'Love is something if you give it away; it comes right back to you'. Try it and see if it works.*
>
> *1 John 4:11*

References

1 Lowen A. *The Language of the Body*. New York: Collier Books; 1958.
2 The UK Osteopathic Information Service. British Osteopathic Association: www.osteopathy.org.uk (accessed 12 October 2006).
3 Williams N, Wilkinson C, Russell I *et al*. Randomised osteopathic manipulation study (ROMANS): pragmatic trial for spinal pain in primary care: *Fam Pract* 2003; 20: 662.
4 Licciardone JC, Brimhall AK and King LN. Osteopathic manipulative treatment for low back pain: a systematic review and meta-analysis randomised controlled trials. *BMC Musculo-skelet Disord* 2005; 6: 43.
5 Parker GB. A controlled trial of cervical manipulation of migraine. *Aust NZ J Med* 1989; 8: 589–93.
6 Klougart N, Nilsson N and Jacobsen J. Infantile colic treated by chiropractors: a prospective study of 316 cases. *J Manip Physiol Ther* 1989; 12: 281–8.
7 Carter B. A pilot study to evaluate the effectiveness of the Bowen technique in management of clients with frozen shoulder. *Complement Ther Med* 2001; 9: 208–15.

Further reading

- Fryman V. Learning difficulties of children viewed in the light of the osteopathic concept. *J Am Osteopath Assoc* 1976; 76: 46–61.
- Hurwitz EL. Manipulation and mobilization of the cervical spine, a systematic review of the literature. *Spine* 1996; 21: 1746–59.

Contacts

- *British Association for Applied Chiropractic*: The Post Office, Cherry Street, Stratton Audley, Nr Bicester OX27 9BA
- *British Chiropractic Association*: www.chiropractic-uk.co.uk; Belgrave House, 17 Belgrave Street, Reading, Berkshire RG1 1QB; tel: 01189 505950
- *British Osteopathic Association*: www.osteopathy.org; Langham House West, Mill Street, Luton, Bedfordshire LU1 2NA; tel: 01582 488455
- *General Osteopathic Council*: www.osteopathy.org.uk; Osteopathy House, 176 Tower Bridge Road, London EC1R 0AA

17

Prayer

Science without Religion is lame
and Religion without science is blind.

Albert Einstein[1]

Prayer, the word, entered the English language via old French *prier*, which comes from the old Latin *precari* 'ask earnestly, beg, pray'; it is an old word for 'pledge' or 'I pray thee'. Prayer is the process of addressing a superhuman being for purposes of praise, adoration, thanksgiving petition or penitence. It does not belong to any particular religion or culture. The basis of prayer differs according to the understanding of God's relationship to humans and their world. In Christian belief, God's concern for humanity is manifested in the incarnation of Jesus Christ who taught his disciples the Lord's Prayer.[2]

Prayer like complementary therapies can also add quality to our spiritual journey. It can be communal, as in public worship it gives a sense of purpose, a means of collective participation in universal cultural themes. This can help as a method of communication and connection to the higher gifts and of divine worship. Prayer is a mode of communication beyond self, within self and through self. It can be used as a mantra for meditation, and it helps to raise lowered energy levels in depression.[3] The physical ritual of prayer can often help relieve anxiety when used as a medium of focus in situations where thinking is difficult. This has a similar effect to a relaxation or breathing technique. Prayer can be invaluable in death and dying and during funeral and burial services for all denominations. It raises the spirits, giving joy and a special meaning to a wedding or baptismal celebration. Prayer is the common language of the faithful and often used as a means of communication with God, which is special, familiar and uplifting for many. When we find ourselves in difficult and hopeless situations it is perhaps the only means of expression that is positive and reassuring. It can be said that, apart from a means of communication with God, regular prayer life can be used as a highly effective tool for health promotion.[4,5]

In a recent statement in a highly respected Catholic journal, on the need for religion, Cardinal George Pell of Sydney, Australia stated that, 'Religion is the antidote to the epidemic of depression in the western world'.[4] He felt that major depression in rich countries was increasing with each generation. At present levels, one in five experience an attack of depression at some time, and three-quarters of a million are seriously depressed each year in Australia. Research showed that African-Caribbean people and Hispanics have less depression in the US than the nearby population of Philadelphia, because of their belief system. Cardinal Pell cited US psychologist Professor Martin Seligman who gave the main reasons for this crisis: an instant pleasure expectation, increased individualism and self-centredness. There is also a heightened sense of victimisation (someone else's fault), an inability to accept that life is tough and failure to learn strategies necessary for survival.

Evidence

In a recent major study in America on the effects of intercessory prayer, 395 men and women in a coronary care unit had received the usual medical care. A number of patients were focused on specifically by prayer groups, others were not; the prayer group did much better than the control group in all aspects of postoperative care.[5]

The latest studies from the Institute of Healthcare research in America also suggest that we might be better off healthwise to attend church than go to the gym. In an analysis of 42 research studies investigating the role of religion in health, 126 000 people were interviewed. It demonstrated that regular attendance at church, synagogue, mosque or Buddhist monastery was significant in prolonging life.[3]

Studies have shown that people who take religion seriously are mentally and physically healthier. They have lower blood pressure, lower incidence of cancer and heart disease, and are significantly less affected by mental health problems. This research also highlighted how long we live, based on participation in religious services, and found higher survival rates in more than 29% of those who participated than in those with no religious involvement.[3] The more we attend religious services, we will effectively suffer less ill-health. Another combined study in America by the same researcher Dr M McCullough, in 21 000 people, reported that those who never attended church had almost twice the risk of death in a nine-year follow-up period. He compared this with those who attended more than once a week and found that it translates into a seven-year difference in life expectancy.[3]

Benefits of prayer and religion

It has been shown that regular church attendance is beneficial for health and longevity.[5,6] Findings are that:

- there is a lower incidence of depression
- people who attend church, mosque, synagogue or monastery services regularly show evidence of greater happiness
- they have lower blood pressure
- they have less incidence of heart disease
- they have lower incidence of cancer
- going to church equates with a longer lifespan
- those who regularly attend church recover faster following surgery
- it prolongs life following heart surgery
- church-goers have better ability to deal with pain
- they have lower stress level
- it improves social interaction
- there is a built-in emotional and spiritual support system
- there is improved ability to deal with stress levels
- there is improved immunity
- church-going is a means of communication in bereavement
- it helps relieve anxiety during the dying process.

There is security and rest in the wisdom of the eternal Scriptures.

James 1:5

References

1 Einstein A. *The World as I See It*. New York: Philosophical Library; 1949.
2 Bradshaw PF. *Daily Prayer in the Early Church*. London: Alcuin Club; 1981.
3 McCullough ME, Hoyt WT and Lanson DB. Religious involvement and mortality: a meta-analytic review. *Health Psychol* 2000; 19: 211–22.
4 Pell G. Too Much Depression. Archdiocese of Sydney [article on website 2006]. www.sydney.catholic.org.au
5 Byrd RC. Positive therapeutic effect of intercessory prayer in a coronary care unit population. *South J Med* 1988; 81: 826–9.
6 O'Laoire S. An experimental study of the effects of distance intercessory prayer on self-esteem, anxiety and depression. *Altern Ther Health Med* 1997; 3: 38–53.

Further reading

• Benson H. *Timeless Healing: the power and biology of belief* (1e). New York: Scribner; 1996.
• Koenig HC and Cohen H. Attendance of religious services, interleukin-6 and other biological indicators of immune function in older adults. *Int J Psychiatry Med* 1997; 23: 233–50.
• Koenig HG, McCullough ME and Lanson DB. *Handbook of Religion and Health* (1e). New York: Oxford University Press; 2001.
• Thompson K. Miracles on demand: prayer and the causation of healing (editorial). *Altern Ther Health Med* 1997; 3: 92–6.

18

Reflexology

To heal our relationship to our bodies is to heal our relationship with the Earth.
To regain our aliveness, and the foundation of all that follows.

Anodea Judith[1]

Reflexology is a physical therapy, a natural hands-on touch technique, a holistic method of treating and preventing illness with foot massage. It is thought that disease of a specific area of the body is matched up with reflex areas mostly found in the hands and feet. It is believed that illness occurs when 'energy channels' in the body are blocked, obstructing the free flow of energy to a specific area.

Feet are thought by reflexology practitioners to represent a 'mirror image' of the body. Equally they are our physical connection to the earth. The left foot represents the left side of the body, and the right foot the right side. It seems rather a simplistic equation, but it has proven to be an effective method of complementary therapy and an ill-health prevention tool. A specific area on the sole of the foot corresponds to a particular organ or area, for example the big toe deals with the head and brain and the little toe the sinuses. The actual foot massage itself is thought to initiate healing because of the touch and subsequent relaxation effect. This method is a drug-free therapy, and no technological gadgetry is required, just a one-to-one relationship with a therapist. It is practised mainly on the feet, but can include the hands, ears, face and back. Sometimes it is called reflex zone therapy, which uses pressure points and energy pathways similar to those in acupressure and acupuncture.

It is thought that illness shows up as a tender spot on the reflex areas of the affected organs and that applying specific foot massage techniques to the corresponding tender spot can help resolve and heal the problem. Almost any area or organ can be treated in this way. Reflexology is a highly refined and sophisticated touch therapy. It is not simply a massage, but offers many other health benefits. Every treatment includes massage of both feet; all the organs are stimulated by using the thumb to apply pressure to the soles. These are examined including the dorsum, medial and lateral aspects of the feet. The therapist is also feeling for tender areas, which correspond to specific areas of an organ that may signify 'imbalance' in that area. Reflexology is not generally used as a diagnostic tool.

History

Reflexology originated in China around 5000 years ago, where it was recognised that there was a link between one part of the body and another, that could be exploited to treat the whole person. The theory is that disease in one part of the body affects the whole organism. Reflexology therapists use charts and maps depicting zones and reflex areas of the soles of the feet, which reflect the body in miniature and are superimposed on a diagram of the foot.

Egyptians used similar methods, which were found on ancient wall paintings found in a tomb in Cairo. In more recent times around 1913 Dr William Fitzgerald, an ear, nose and throat (ENT) surgeon, divided the body into 10 zones or channels. He maintained that vital energy flowed through these channels from the toes to the head, hands and back, covering all organs and areas of the body. Dr Fitzgerald is widely acknowledged as the founder of this zone or channel version of modern reflexology. Even in the early days of integration he worked in conjunction with many other health professionals, osteopaths, doctors and dentists.

By the 1930s, an American lady, Eunice Ingham refined and devised the present system of reflexology where the therapist used thumbs to massage the soles of the feet on specific pressure points. She wrote and published two books *Stories the Feet can Tell Them. Reflexology* and *Stories the Feet have Told Them. Reflexology*.[2,3] She was known as the matriarch of western reflexology. The first reflexology clinic in Britain was established in the 1960s by Doreen Bayley, and reflexology has since become a very popular form of holistic health care.

Benefits of reflexology

The benefits of reflexology are thought to be psychological, physiological and spiritual. The one-to-one relationship has a highly valued effect, and continuity of care brings its own benefits and rewards. It is thought to have a relaxation effect, increasing feelings of being more positive and improving sleep patterns. This therapy also helps stimulate the body's own ability to heal and defend itself. It offers pain relief, reducing the need for drugs. A therapist can identify areas of the body that are going through 'negative' change due to possible ill-health.

Evidence

Research on healthy volunteers has demonstrated, via ultrasound, the physical effects of reflexology, with a definite change in renal flow in the body.[4] Studies have also shown encouraging results, which included the relationship of client and therapist, possibly adding to the placebo effect. It is believed that the analgesic effect is achieved through 'blocking' the nerves. This is based on the same principle as transcutaneous electrical nerve stimulation (TENS), and is thought to suppress and relax pain impulses. It may also work by stimulating the release of hormones that are beneficial for health, such as endorphins, the body's natural pain relievers and mood enhancers.[5,6]

The foot can reveal the psychological state of the individual as well as the personality traits. It is thought that each foot reflects different qualities of the person, be they creative, practical, masculine or feminine, and determines who is at risk of ill-health given a specific type of personality.

Reflexology is one of the major integrated therapies that was included in an investigation of the use of complementary therapies within the UK pain clinics, the Pain Audit Collection System (PACS) which is a database set up in 1987 by the Pain Society.[7]

Chronic pain is a multidimensional issue most effectively treated using an inter-disciplinary approach. The use of complementary therapies is becoming an increasingly acceptable health behaviour in the UK. A postal survey found that 50% of chronic pain patients had used complementary therapies. Most complementary therapies are provided outside the NHS, and 77% of chronic pain patients were self-referred.[7] Studies have also shown that reflexology is effective in the relief of pain in cancer care.[8] This therapy is firmly established as an effective complementary tool for health care and is well integrated into mainstream services. Many nurses, physiotherapists and health visitors use reflexology within the NHS.

Conditions where reflexology is beneficial

- Asthma
- Arthritis
- Anxiety
- Hypertension
- Back and neck pain
- Migraines
- Musculoskeletal conditions
- Rheumatism
- Sinus problems
- Palliative care
- Premenstrual syndrome
- Menopause
- Stress
- Chronic disease

We don't see things as they are. We see things as we are.

Anaïs Nin

References

1 Judith A. *Eastern Body, Western Mind*. Berkeley, CA: Celestial Arts; 1996.
2 Ingham E. *The Original Works of Eunice D Ingham: Stories the Feet can Tell Them. Reflexology and Stories the Feet have Told Them. Reflexology*. St Petersburg: Ingham Publishing Inc; 1984.
3 Adamson S, Harris E and Kerr S. *The Reflexology Partnership*. London: Kyle Cathie; 1995.
4 Sudmeier I, Bodner G, Egger I *et al*. Changes of the renal blood flow during organ-associated foot reflexology measured by colour Doppler sonography. *Forsch Komplementarmed* 1999; 6: 129–34.
5 Melzack R and Wall PD. Pain mechanisms: a new theory. *Science* 1965; 150: 971–9.
6 Lett A. *Reflex Zone Therapy for Health Professionals*. London: Churchill Livingstone; 2000.
7 Rice I, Price C and Bryant T. The use of complementary therapies within UK pain clinics. In: Darnell D, Pinder M and Treacy K (eds). *Searching for Evidence: complementary therapies research*. London: The Prince of Wales Foundation for Integrated Health; 2006; pp. 51–2.
8 Stephenson N. *The Effects and Duration of Foot Reflexology on Pain in Patients with Metastatic Cancer*. North Carolina: East Carolina University; 2006.

Further reading

- Mackereth PA, Tiran D (eds). *Clinical Reflexology*. London: Churchill Livingstone; 2005.
- Trousdell P. Reflexology meets emotional needs. *Int J Altern Complement Med* 1996; November: 9–12.

Contacts

- *The Association of Reflexologists*: www.reflexology.org/aor; 27 Old Gloucester Street, London WC1 3XX; tel: 0870 567 3320
- *Reflexions*: www.aor.org.uk

Reiki

*Until we know the state of your inner harmony, we can at the most release you
from your illness because your inner harmony is the source of your health. But
when we release you from one illness, you will immediately catch another
because nothing has been done with regard to your inner harmony. The fact of
the matter is that it is your inner harmony which must be supported.*

Paracelsus

Reiki was discovered and developed by a Doctor Mikao Usui who was born in Japan
in 1865. This is an ancient healing method, which has become very popular here in
the west. Reiki is a very practical energy-healing technique that is easy to learn and
easy to use. Anyone who has an open mind with an interest in holism and healing
can learn to harness the healing powers of the earth's energy. It provides a 'hands-
on' approach to relaxation and healing, and is a source of enrichment to everyday
life.

The word Reiki means 'universal life force energy', *rei*, pronounced ('rey')
describes the universal aspect of the energy and *ki* ('kee') is the life force energy
that flows through all living things. Many ancient cultures have handed down
knowledge of hands-on healing methods throughout history and referred to the
universal life force energy to promote 'wellbeing'. This is known as *qi* by the
Chinese, *prana* by the Hindus, *baraka* by the Sufis, *ka* by the ancient Egyptians and
light by Christians.[1]

History

The secrets of these ancient healing traditions were closely guarded and were only
passed on to the privileged few by word of mouth, usually to priests, spiritual
healers and Sufis. Dr Usui's years of research led to the discovery of this healing art
form towards the end of the 19th century. He continued to develop and eventually
began to teach and pass on the knowledge of energy healing by the early 1920s, to a
Dr Hayashi. He subsequently founded a clinic in Tokyo. In Hawaii, in 1935, a Reiki
clinic was established, by a Japanese/American, Mrs Hayayo Takata, who had
suffered from depression and decided to try Reiki energy healing.[2] She trained and
became a master practitioner and worked very successfully using this method for
the next 40 years. In the 1970s she passed on her techniques to over 20 masters, and
today the same techniques are being taught and developed here in the west.

*There are only two ways to live your life, one is as though nothing is a miracle the
other is as if everything is a miracle.*

Albert Einstein[3]

We as humans can only find happiness in all aspects of life in the present moment. If the best part of our attention is focused on the past or the future, we find it more difficult to learn from and deal with life's challenges. People who generally live in the present have a clearer view of life events and feel less threatened and challenged. Reiki energy goes some way to help focus the mind, body and spirit to the present, awakening its potential harmony with the universe.

Benefits of Reiki

- Develops conscious awareness.
- Helps with pain reduction.
- Relieves physical tension.
- Helps to make decisions from a balanced perspective.
- Promotes relaxation and restful sleep.
- Balances negative thoughts that stop our development.
- Creates an awareness of positive and negative patterns.
- Releases repressed feelings and emotions.
- Generates a feeling of courage and confidence to face life.
- Creates feelings of peace, relaxation and security.
- Helps make connections between negative attitudes and thoughts and physical illness.
- Promotes the regeneration of low energy levels, particularly in depression.
- Integrates fully with other forms of health care.

Reiki can also be used in first aid, for example, in bleeding to stem the flow and to relieve pain to calm the nervous system.[4] A person can receive an immediate experience of the divine. It can be used before and after operations to promote healing. Reiki can never be a substitute for conventional medical care, but can be very effective as a complementary tool. There is no personal energy 'drained' from the therapist. Care must be taken with people who have a pacemaker or suffer with mania. In these instances a medical opinion is essential.

> *Life is a song – sing it*
> *Life is a game – play it*
> *Life is a challenge – meet it*
> *Life is a dream – realise it*
> *Life is a sacrifice – offer it*
> *Life is love – enjoy it.*
>
> *Sai Baba*[5]

A Reiki treatment session

Reiki energy is thought by its many practitioners to be a gift from the universe and available to everyone. The body consists of seven main energy centres or *chakras*, from the Sanskrit meaning 'wheel'. Each corresponds with the regions and organs of the endocrine system. Hands placed over the body direct this cosmic energy through the *chakras* during the course of a Reiki treatment.

The practicalities of a Reiki session

This is basically a procedure that harnesses the energy that surrounds all living matter and channels it to good use for the needs of the human condition.

Ideally it should take place in a warm quiet room with calming music and candlelight.

- The client should be on a chair, bed or treatment couch.
- The client should preferably be fully clothed, flat on their back, covered with a blanket.
- The therapist's hands are placed on various parts of the body from the top of the client's head to the feet and then on to the back.
- A session will last about 45 minutes.
- A client must drink plenty of water before and after the treatment.
- A person may experience warmth, crying, tingling, laughter, vibrations, sleepiness, or may see colours during the session.
- There should be one session weekly for 4–6 weeks, depending on the client's progress.
- It is advisable not to drive long distances or operate machinery following a Reiki session.

Medical conditions where Reiki is beneficial

- Anxiety
- Depression
- Stress
- Insomnia
- Palliative care
- Musculoskeletal conditions
- Headaches
- Menopause
- Premenstrual and menstrual problems
- Irritable bowel syndrome
- In pain relief
- Chronic disease management and prevention

References

1 Lubeck W, Petter FA and Rand W. *The Spirit of Reiki*. Twin Lakes, WI: Lotus Press, Shangri-La; 2001.
2 Brown F. *Living Reiki, Takata's Teachings*. Mendocino, CA: Life Rhythm; 1992.
3 Einstein A. *The World as I See It*. New York: Philosophical Library; 1949.
4 Lubeck W. *Reiki for First Aid*. Twin Lakes, WI: Lotus Light, Shangri-La; 1995.
5 Ruhela SP. *Sri Sathya Sai Baba: Life and Divine Role*. New Delhi: Vikas; 1993.

Further reading

- Chopra D. *Boundless Energy*. London: Rider Books; 1995.

- Kumar R. *Kundalini for Beginners*. Minnesota: Llewellyn Publications; 2000.
- Oshmann J. *Energy Medicine – The Scientific Basis*. Edinburgh: Churchill Livingstone; 2000.
- Parkes C and Parkes P. *Reiki. The essential guide to the ancient healing art*. London: Vermillion; 1998.
- Thornton L. A study of Reiki: an energy treatment using Roger's science. *Rogerian Nurs Sci News* 1996; 8: 14–15.

Contacts

- *The Reiki Association*: www.reikiassociation.org.uk; 2 Manor Cottages, Stockley Hill, Peterchurch, Hereford HR2 0SS; tel: 01981 550829
- *The Reiki School Budworth*: Shay Lane, Hale, Altrincham, Cheshire WA15 8UE; tel: 0161 980 6453

20

Traditional Chinese medicine

All the tragedy in the world, in the individual and in the multitude, comes from lack of harmony. And harmony is best given by producing harmony in one's own life.

Hazrat Inayat Khan[1]

Traditional Chinese medicine (TCM) is a total and complete system of health care, and a form of preventive medicine. It is a unique combination of holistic principles that leads to diagnosis and cure of illness, which has been practised in China for thousands of years. The oriental approach is still practised in China and is well integrated with the more conventional western style of health care, but is fundamentally different from that of western medicine. In TCM, an understanding of the human body is based on the theory that the body as a whole organism and the planet are inextricably linked. Historically, TCM combined herbal and plant medicine, massage, acupuncture, qigong (breathing and meditation exercises), Tai Chi (Chinese martial arts) and Feng Shui (Chinese astrology). This also encompassed a spiritual relationship with the environment, earth and universe. At present it is more fragmented and focuses mainly on Chinese herbal medicine and acupuncture, with the addition of massage and meditation.

History and philosophy

The principle of TCM is to assist the body to regain balance and achieve harmony. Practitioners believe that there is not a **single** cause or **factor** that creates ill-health nor that there is a **single** cure. This approach encompasses the whole body and its constitutional type of personality and the environmental conditions, such as heat, dampness, cold and wind. The oriental philosophy maintains that the body is thought of as a whole (internal) organism, and includes a relationship to its (external) environment, which is crucial for balance. Human energy is known as *qi*, which is influenced by outside environmental factors. Personal energy is supported by a positive and healthy approach to lifestyle – this includes a balanced diet, exercise, rest and relaxation. Low energy levels, as a result of personal abuse, neglect or excess, are thought to deplete energy that is essential for a healthy functioning body.

Therapists believe that *yin* (inactive qualities), *yang* (active qualities) and the five elements of the earth have to work in harmony for the desired effect for positive good health. This is achieved partly by tension, created by opposites, for example male and female, light and dark, hot and cold, thus creating energy and movement that flows freely through living cells. *Yin* is inactive and internal, which is cold, dark and descending. *Yang* is external, hot, bright and ascending. The energy, with the *yin* and *yang* balance, should flow freely through the many pathways and channels of the body, creating a homeostasis. The process is also helped by the relationship between the physical body and its environment. This includes wood, fire, earth, water and metal, which are linked to the circulatory pathways. These elements are used to interpret the relationship between the physiology and pathology of the human body and its natural environment. They explain the connection between material objects as well as the unity between the body and the natural world. The theory is that wood promotes fire, fire promotes earth, earth promotes metal, metal promotes water and water generates wood. This is a circular and endless promotion of different elements maintaining a natural balance of the body as a multisensory organism.

Evidence

A controlled trial of traditional Chinese medical herbs in widespread non-exudative atopic eczema proved very successful with encouraging results.[2] An 18 months' follow-up trial of children treated with Chinese herbal medicine for atopic eczema showed significant improvement in 60% of cases.[3] Equally, adults with eczema showed significant improvement.[4] Studies have also shown positive effects in irritable bowel syndrome.[5]

Chinese herbal medicines are not suitable for self-medication.

Most of the remedies are not prescribed or sold as single herbs but in complex compounds and varied combinations. There is little research available so it is difficult to evaluate efficacy. Chinese massage and acupuncture are considered safe and well documented. Therefore for safety reasons, Chinese herbal medicine should only be prescribed by a qualified registered practitioner. This complex subject requires years of training and expertise. These mixtures can cause adverse effects such as allergic reactions, liver damage and renal failure. Chinese herbal combinations are not regulated in the same way as nutritional supplements in the UK. There is also a risk of herb substitution with unknown substances. The adulteration with chemicals, inappropriate dosage and misuse in general, can easily lead to accidental poisoning. TCM is not regulated in the UK but there is a register (*see* Contacts, p. 110). The requirement is a minimum of five years' training, including three years' training in western medicine.

Medical applications of traditional Chinese medicine

- Asthma
- Eczema, dermatitis
- Menstrual problems, premenstrual syndrome
- Menopause
- Immune system support
- Chronic fatigue
- Side-effects of chemotherapy
- Digestive disorders
- Drug addiction withdrawal
- Prostate cancer (as complementary treatment)

Caution in the use of herbal mixtures and compounds

As in all medical practice, caution is needed in the use of herbs and drugs in pregnancy, and an awareness of drug interactions, for example with the contraceptive pill, anticoagulant, antihypertensive and heart medication. Special precaution is advised in diabetes mellitus and bleeding diatheses. Many patients who consult herbal practitioners are unaware of this information.

> *Take one day at a time, God gives just enough light to see the next step and that's all we need.*
>
> *Psalms 27:1*

References

1 Khan PZI (ed). *A Pearl in Wine: Essays in the Life, Music and Sufism of Hazrat Inayat Khan*. New Lebanon, NY: Omega; 2001.
2 Sheehan MP and Atherton DJ. A controlled trial of traditional Chinese medical herbs in widespread non-exudative atopic eczema. *Br J Dermatol* 1992; 126: 179–84.
3 Sheehan MP and Atherton DJ. One-year follow up of children with Chinese medical herbs for atopic eczema. *Br J Dermatol* 1994; 130: 488–93.
4 Sheehan MP and Atherton DJ. Efficacy of traditional Chinese herbal therapy in adult atopic dermatitis. *Lancet* 1992; 340: 13–17.
5 Bensoussan A, Talley NJ, Hing M et al. Treatment of irritable bowel syndrome with Chinese herbal medicine: a randomized controlled trial. *JAMA* 1998; 280: 1585–9.

Further reading

- Holland A. *Voices of Qi. An introductory guide to traditional Chinese medicine*. Berkeley, CA: North Atlantic Books; 2000.
- Maciocia G. *The Foundations of Chinese Medicine. A comprehensive text for acupuncturists and herbalists*. London: Churchill Livingstone; 2005.
- Unschuld PU. *Medicine in China: a history of ideas*. Berkeley, CA: University of California Press; 1985.

Contacts

- *Traditional Chinese Medicine, Register of Chinese Herbal Medicine*: www.rchm.co.uk; 11–15 Betterton Street, London WC2H 9BP; tel: 020 7470 8740
- *Merging Chinese Traditional Medicine into the American Health System*: www.jyi.org
- *Journal of Chinese Medicine*: www.jcm.co.uk

21

Yoga

Yoga is an experience, not a system of thought; it is to be lived, not intellectually analysed. To achieve this, meditation is indispensable.

Richard Hittleman[1]

Yoga is known universally as a health-enhancement tool, used in conjunction with meditation. It is a practical, non-religious form of mental and physical exercise used the world over by Christians, atheists, Jews, Muslims and Buddhists. Yoga philosophy accepts the body as a vehicle or vessel for the soul on its journey towards enlightenment. Master yogi of the east and west believe 'know thy self' and therein lies the answer to the universal riddle of life, death, leading to peace of mind, body and spirit.[2]

Yoga in the complementary field of medicine is described as a 'well-rounded', holistic therapy. This approach allows the individual to take personal responsibility for health, of mind, body and breath, ultimately taking control of their life. It is usually combined with meditation and it is this combination that makes it such a unique, holistic, and all-round discipline, for the enhancement of wellbeing.[2,3] As a result of yoga's increasing popularity, influences can be seen in today's fashions in television and advertising. As a result of this exposure, many people are interested in how to include yoga in their treatment plans for disease management. Many institutions sponsor yoga classes regularly, including the workplace. It can be practised alone or in a group, and promotes social interaction. Physically, it is considered a low-impact activity, so people of all ages and sizes, shapes and conditions can participate in the practice of yoga.[3] This holistic and unique therapy can be used as a very useful tool for health promotion and in prevention of ill-health.

History and philosophy

Historically, yoga was practised in India about 5000 years ago. It is based on the tenets of simple living and high thinking. Great sages (wise, discreet, judicious people) practised yoga regularly, and in doing so felt a connection with nature, realising that energy flows through all forms of life. From this knowledge, skills were honed and developed to direct energy to body parts for greater physical and emotional health awareness. The aim of the yogi is eventual liberation that results from self-realisation and knowledge.[3]

The Sanskrit translation of yoga, *yuj*, means to yoke together, or a union of the mind and body, to make whole. Yoga in the west is practised in many forms, although Hatha yoga is the type we are most familiar with that includes physical postures. The sanskrit *ha* means sun or positive aspects, and *tha* means moon or negative aspects It represents the relationship of opposites, such as dark to light, male to female, and yin and yang. Hatha yoga seeks to unite polarities and resolve conflicts into a state of balance of union and harmony. Most of the knowledge and history relating to yoga has come from ancient texts, the *Vedas*, the *Upanishads*, the *Bhagavad Gita* and the *Yoga Sutras*.

The Vedas (knowledge)

These are the Hindu scriptures from around the second century AD and are the oldest written tradition in India. They explore the possibility of the human spirit and discuss the purpose and meaning of life.

The Upanishads

This translates as 'to sit down close to one's teachers'. They are writings dating as far back as the middle of the second millennium and are philosophical poems that explore the nature of the universal soul.

The Bhagavad Gita (The Lord's song)

This comes from the third or fourth century BC and is written as a dialogue between Lord Krishna and his devotee Arjuna on the battle of good and evil in all of mankind. It also explores the various yogic paths to liberation.

The Yoga Sutras (aphorisms on yoga)

These are philosophical writings from around the second century BC and are on techniques for spiritual growth and development. Most modern yogis regard it as the authority on yoga. It includes the eight-fold path of yoga.[4]
There are many other types of yoga including:

- *Raga yoga*: the way to balance and union through meditation and control of the mind
- *Jnana yoga*: knowledge or study
- *Bhakti yoga*: about devotion and selfless love
- *Karma yoga*: wholeness through action, service and work
- *Mantra yoga*: union through sound vibration and speech.

A yoga session

A Hatha yoga (this is the most commonly practised form of yoga in the west) session consists of:

- *meditation*: creates an inner connection and improves concentration to help focus the mind
- *breath control*: helps regulate breathing and oxygenation of the blood, and clears the body of waste products such as carbon dioxide
- *postures*: increase blood flow to specific organs and increase flexibility
- *affirmation and visualisation* (optional): helps concentrate energy on a particular area of the body and reconditions the unconscious mind
- *meditation*: creates peace of mind and reconnects to the present.

The benefits of yoga

- Helps calms the mind.
- Integrates the mental and physical.
- Creates a positive mind set.
- Frees the mind.
- Creates self-awareness.
- Aids stress reduction.
- Is a tool for enlightenment.

By using a mind/body approach to ill health, prevention and health care we can alter every aspect of our physiological and mental functioning. We can also gain self-knowledge, physical grace and spiritual freedom.

Applications in modern medicine

- Anxiety
- Depression
- Asthma
- Circulation problems
- Insomnia
- Premenstrual syndrome
- Pain relief
- Stress
- Irritable bowel syndrome
- Bereavement
- Menopause
- Weight reduction
- Management of chronic illness
- Palliative care

> *It's good to have a daily quiet time, an opportunity to give God time to speak to our lives as we meditate on his Word.*
>
> *Psalms 19:14*
> *Psalms 46:10*

Reference

1 Hittleman R. *Guide to Yoga Meditation*. New York: Bantam Books; 1969.
2 La Forge R. Mind body fitness, encouraging prospects for primary and secondary prevention. *J Cardiovasc Nurs* 1997; 11: 53–65.
3 Hoenig J. Medical research of yoga. *Confin Pschiatr* 1968; 11: 69–89.
4 Feuerstein G. *The Yoga Sutra of Pantanjali*. Rochester: VT Inner Traditions; 1979.

Further reading

- Benson H. *The Relaxation Response*. New York: Avon Books; 1975.
- Keleman S. *Your Body Speaks its Mind*. USA: Centre Press; 1975.
- Lasator J. *Relax and Renew, Restful Yoga for Stressful Times*. London: Rodwell Press; 1992.

- Neinstraub M. *Alternative and Complementary Treatment in Neurolgic Illness*. London: Churchill Livingstone; 2001.
- Weller S. *Yoga Therapy*. London: HarperCollins; 1995.

Contacts

- *British Wheel of Yoga*: 25 Jermyn Street, Sleaford, Lincolnshire; tel: 01529 306 851
- *Sivanada Yoga*: Venanta Centre, 51 Felsham Road, London SW15 1AZ; tel: 0181 780–0160
- *Yoga for Health Foundation*: www.yogaforhealthfoundation.co.uk; Ickwell Bury, Ickwell Green, Biggleswade SG18 9EF; tel: 01767 627271

22

Health and lifestyle

In order to develop love – universal love, cosmic love, whatever you would like to call it – one must accept the whole situation of life as it is, both the light and the dark, the good and the bad.

Chogyam Trungpa[1]

A positive approach to a balanced lifestyle promotes 'wellbeing' and prevents ill-health in the longer term. It is not about the length of our lives, but the quality of that life in mind, body and spirit. A good life requires balance and moderation in all aspects for the ultimate achievement of optimum health. It is a combination of physical, emotional, psychological and spiritual endeavours in order to achieve our goal. A healthy balanced mind generally has a positive attitude to lifestyle and takes responsibility for the standard of nutritional input, physical activity, rest, relaxation and general health care.

This chapter deals with nutritional medicine, exercise, relaxation, music and spiritual health, and serves as a reminder of our fundamental needs. If we obtain the balance, through integration of these requirements it may well form a sound basis for health promotion. Conventional medicine, with all its up-to-date technology, focuses very much on disease and on the scientific treatments and cures. The word 'medicine' comes from the Latin *medico*, meaning drug. Surgical intervention and drugs such as antidepressants, antibiotics and analgesics form the mainstay of modern medicine. For these amazing advances we are more than grateful because they save lives, relieve pain and replace deficiencies. Treatment and support are very much someone else's responsibility, with this model of care. Specialisation in the medical and scientific worlds unfortunately helps to distort the bigger picture in terms of health of the whole organism. People can easily become defined by body parts, which in a practical sense increases efficiency and cultivates greater skills in specific areas, for example the heart, lungs, kidneys and intestines both large and small. The responsibility, therefore, in caring for the rest of the human condition is left to the individual's choice. This can lead to confusion in terms of which pathway to take or what therapy to use for an individual's particular needs.

Positive good health and the prevention of ill-health are an individual's responsibilities and require an active input, effort and determination. It is part of our journey, and the older we get the more obvious and precious the quality of that life becomes. It cannot be taken for granted. The feelings of peace, harmony and contentment in a lifetime are short-lived and are more precious with hindsight. We only truly appreciate good health when we, or a member of our family or close friends, have been affected by ill-health.

Poverty brings its own hardship and difficulties, with poor housing, increased tendency to smoke cigarettes, higher alcohol intake and diet of greater carbohydrate content. Energy is invested more in terms of survival than in health promotion or in long-term prevention of ill-health. Added to this, there is a tendency to use illegal drugs and a higher use of prescription drugs. These conditions are not conducive to fostering and achieving positive health.

In order to keep up with the demands of a hectic lifestyle, we tend to over-indulge in the use of stimulants to help support the stressed immune system. Alcohol, nicotine, caffeine and drugs are used regularly to help us get through the day. Unfortunately these have adverse effects and can result in long-term addiction. Achieving and maintaining better health 'with the perfect body' has become a modern-day prescription. The vast majority of purchases over the counter are in general a search for the prevention of common ailments, to slow down the aging process, or provide nutritional supplements and natural means to induce sleep and relaxation. Most common illnesses are self-limiting and require reassurance rather than medical interventions.

Nutritional medicine

A clinical review in the *BMJ* in 1999 reported:

> *Although nutrition, as a science, has always been part of conventional medicine, doctors are not taught, and therefore do not practise, much in the way of nutritional therapies. Dieticians in conventional settings, tend to work mainly with particular patients, such as those with diabetes, obesity, digestive and swallowing problems, or cardiovascular risk factors. Apart from the treatment of gross nutritional deficiencies and rare metabolic disorders, other nutritional interventions generally fall outside the mainstream and can therefore be described as complementary medicine.*[2,3]

Existing health problems where nutritional management is helpful

There are many conditions where a dietary review and change of habit will relieve symptoms and improve 'wellbeing':

- insomnia
- asthma
- arthritis
- alcohol and drug dependency
- anaemia
- anxiety
- Crohn's disease
- cancers
- bulimia
- anorexia nervosa
- dyspepsia
- eczema, psoriasis
- infertility
- irritable bowel syndrome
- diabetes
- breast feeding
- pregnancy
- depression, dementia

- infections
- ulcerative colitis
- hyperactive and learning difficulties in children
- the elderly
- osteoporosis
- migraine, headaches
- candida infections
- heart disease
- coeliac disease
- compromised immune system
- stress
- allergies
- preconceptual care
- menopause
- prescribed medication such as the contraceptive pill and antibiotics

Common nutritional supplements

- Multivitamins and minerals for general health care
- Evening primrose oil, for PMS and atopic dermatitis
- Vitamin B_6 (pyridoxine) for morning sickness and PMS
- Garlic for lowering cardiovascular risk
- High-dose vitamin C for cancer
- Zinc for prevention of common colds
- High-dose vitamin for learning disability (orthomolecular therapy)
- Calcium for osteoporosis
- Fish oils, Omega 3 for lowering cardiovascular risk[4]

Professor John Yudkin in the *Journal of Human Nutrition* in 1951 said:

> *I make no apology for saying that the health of the majority of human beings depends more on their nutrition than it does on any other single factor. However important and dramatic have been the advances in hygiene, medicine and surgery, it is still true that even more important will be the effects proper nutrition would have on human morbidity and mortality. For this reason, I believe that the ultimate objective of nutritionists must be the nutritional education of the public.[5]*

Nutritional needs

- Eat a well-balanced diet (as fresh and near natural as possible).
- Be aware of fat intake.
- Be aware of sugar intake.
- Increase fibre intake (at least five portions of fruit and vegetables daily).
- Make sure vitamin C and B complex and mineral intake is adequate.
- Always eat breakfast.
- Drink at least 2 litres of fluid daily.
- Avoid processed food where possible.
- Be aware of salt intake, flavour food with herbs and spices.
- Reduce tea, coffee and alcohol intake.

- Avoid additives, pesticides and insecticides.
- Be aware of red meat intake.
- Increase intake of white meat and fresh fish.
- Good-quality fresh food is essential.
- Be aware of quantity of intake.

There are many factors to be considered when thinking in terms of a balanced diet for the individual, for example, the patient's psychological state, genetic make-up, physical illness and degree of activity. Medication, poverty and allergies are also a consideration. We must remember that pregnancy, breast feeding, age and sex of the individual are all important factors.

Exercise

> *The Body is the Angel of the soul.*
>
> *John O'Donohue[6]*

We cannot expect to be healthy and balanced without regular physical activity. Our body is at risk if we remain inactive. It should be a priority and an individual responsibility, as a basic requirement for ill-health prevention and a way of life. This is an age of physical inactivity, resulting in chronic ill-health such as heart disease and obesity. Good health and fitness are inextricably linked to disease prevention. Physical inactivity is recognised as a risk factor for coronary artery disease. Exercise plays a role in primary and secondary prevention and can also control blood lipid abnormalities, diabetes and obesity. In addition, aerobic exercise adds an independent blood pressure-lowering effect in certain hypertensive groups.[7] Statistics show an alarming rise in obesity in children and young adults, with resulting health risks.[8] Children learn from parental example, so it is good practice to encourage adults to take physical activity and exercise more seriously. Fitness regimes must be tailored to meet the individual's needs, personality, abilities and medical conditions.

Physical exercise could be as simple as a daily walk, and need not necessarily incur any great expense. The benefits are cumulative over a period of time, with sustained input. It should be an enjoyable activity, participated in as an individual, family or group. There is an abundance of different activities in the community for all levels of skill and fitness; exercise does not have to be a chore or practised in isolation.

The benefits of regular exercise

- Mood enhancement, in depression
- Helps balance anxiety levels, focusing on the positive
- Interactive, fun and reduces isolation
- Sense of achievement
- Lowers blood pressure, if only by weight reduction
- Helps regulate sleep pattern, insomnia
- Stabilises weight and aids in weight reduction
- Reduces the incidence of heart disease
- Improves confidence

- Improves flexibility, muscles, ligament and joints
- Aids the elimination of body waste
- Helps massage internal organs
- Enhances the 'feel good factor'
- Gives an example for children to follow

Relaxation

To truly keep our balance it is essential to learn the art of relaxation, by whatever means suitable for the individual needs. Practising the art of relaxing and acquiring the desired goal is actually quite difficult to achieve for the overactive mind. In order to recharge energy levels to allow the body to function at optimum level it is necessary to be proactive. Relaxation can be achieved in many ways, for example through practising yoga or meditation, listening to music or gardening to name but a few. The reduction in sympathetic nerve stimulation is often only made possible by relaxation techniques, which have the benefit of allowing the body to rest and recharge the energy levels in a very structured and direct way. The use of the 24 hour clock of **8 hours' work, 8 hours' relaxation resulting in 8 hours' sleep,** will always help to achieve and maintain a physical and emotional balance. Coping abilities will increase and the individual is more likely to have 'positive' stress experiences, resulting in a feeling of 'wellbeing'.

Muscle relaxation technique

(15 to 20 minutes)
This exercise is devised for **total body relaxation** and generated to focus the mind and at the same time to de-stress and slow down mental activity.

- Sit in a comfortable position in a chair, back supported, both feet flat on the floor, slightly apart. Rest arms in the lap, keep the head straight with the chin parallel to the floor. Breathe from the abdomen and the diaphragm, relax slowly and gently.
- With the eyes closed, direct attention to each part of the body in turn. Each time tense and relax the muscles and concentrate on the sensation of tension and relaxation. Notice that the tension disappears and muscles feel at ease, warm and heavy (take about 10 seconds to relax, 5 seconds to tense).
- Concentrate on the right leg; focus on each part of the leg in turn, starting with the toes. Tense and relax each set of muscles, feel the tension drain away and notice the sensation of heaviness and warmth. Now do the same with the instep, heel and ankle, tense the muscles for 5 seconds and now relax for 10 seconds and feel the relaxation of the limb. Now relax the knee, thigh, and hips, using tension for 5 seconds and now relax for 10 seconds.
- Repeat this exercise with the left leg, starting with the toes, instep and ankle, followed by the knee, thigh and hip.
- Now concentrate on the right arm, starting with the fingers, tense the fingers and thumb for 5 seconds, then relax for about 10 seconds. Do the same with the palm, wrist, forearms, elbow, upper arm and lastly the shoulder; tense and relax each in turn, feel the warmth and heavy sensation.

- Repeat with the left arm, starting with the fingers, tense and relax each part as before, enjoy the relaxed feel of the warm, heavy arm.
- Next the abdominal muscles: pull the middle in tightly, make the waist as small as possible, hold for 5 seconds and relax for 10 seconds.
- Concentrate on the base of the spine, then the rest of the spine, gradually up to the shoulders, tensing and relaxing, feel the spine sink into the chair.
- Now tense and relax the shoulders, feel the tension, then relax, let them drop and feel the relaxation.
- Tense and relax the neck muscles in the same way, keep the head straight and chin parallel to the floor, the head should now be balanced upon the spine.
- Focus the attention on the head. Tense and relax the jaw, let it drop and feel the mouth slightly open, 5 seconds' tension and 10 seconds for relaxation. Tense the tongue, then the eyes, the same rhythmic tension and relaxation. Tense and relax the forehead, notice the relaxation effect of heaviness and warmth.
- Concentrate on the breathing, feel the abdominal muscles move slowly **out** and **up** on the in breath and **down** and **inward** on the out breath. Breathing should be slow, measured and gentle.
- Quieten the mind, allow the thoughts to drift through the head without following them, let them just come and go. Take the mind to a lovely place such as a mountain, woods, or seaside, picture a walk along the seashore, seeing the waves the sand and the sun dancing on the water.
- Sit quietly for 5 minutes, enjoy this state of complete relaxation, the body warm and heavy and relaxed.
- After 5 minutes open the eyes slowly and be aware of the surroundings, in a relaxed state of mind and body.

Music

Music is the cry of the soul. It is a revelation, a thing to be revered. Performances of great musical works are for us what the rites and festivals of religion were to the ancients – an invitation into the mysteries of the human soul.

Frederick Delius (1862–1934)

Music has always had a profound and magical effect on our entire system. It can fill us with joy or move us to tears in an instant. Music inspires movement and rhythmic connections, to calm or excite, and provides entertainment for the mind and food for the soul. We are all deeply affected by sound in some way, be it relaxing, rhythmic or thunderous and energetic. Music therapy is invaluable, a way to express a range of emotions that is too difficult to put into words.[9,10] Music is beneficial in both physical and emotional disabilities. It is particularly therapeutic in autism, children with learning difficulties and for psychogeriatric patients.[9] Songs and music are likened to the spiritual record of humanity in all its guises. Music is often associated with young people, the spirit is awakened by the profound effect of music, changing perspective on their reality. Musical expression is also a major part of religious services and helps bring communities together. The power of sound has long been recognised by spiritual and mystical traditions. In the east for thousands of years, meditation and spiritual exercises have been based on sound, by Buddhist and Islamic traditions in particular. In the west, prayers, chanting and singing hymns in church are an integral part of services, helping to make spiritual connections.

A Swiss scientist Dr Hans Jenny (1904–1972) developed a 'tono-scope' that can depict any sound as a three-dimensional image. It is believed that the sound 'O' made by the human voice produces a perfect sphere creating vibrations.[10] It is thought that the basis of the 'om' or 'aum' (sounds used by Eastern traditions), as well as the Christian and Jewish Amen, is to produce a particular vibrational and rhythmic pattern. These are thought to alter the brain waves in a similar way to relaxation, heightening awareness.[11–12]

Spiritual health

> To lose our connection with the body is to become spiritually homeless, without an anchor, we float aimlessly, battered by the winds and waves of life.
>
> *Anodea Judith*[13]

Spiritual health is perhaps the most important aspect of physical health and mental wholeness. To get the most out of our time on earth it is important that we use all the power available to us. This will help us become anchored to the earth by the 'physical body' and connected to the divine spirit within, by faith through our unique multisensory capabilities of perception.[12] It does not necessarily mean we have to follow a particular religious philosophy to achieve this.

Losing our way through illness, neglect, being misguided or lost can distort the rhythm and normal flow of energy. We can become disassociated from our own personal awareness, losing sight of our inner guiding light and the path to wholeness. A holistic approach to health care places a large emphasis on the individual taking responsibility for their own needs as part of their personal journey. Following this path is an ongoing process. We are not necessarily always aware at a conscious level, it may simply be an instinct. It may perhaps be a feeling of inner knowing or awareness. Each and every one of us has a spiritual path to follow; it is simply a question of choice and connection. For many people, it is through illness, loss or trauma that the reconnection to the divine is made, and the meaning of life discovered through health experience.[11] People who have never become disconnected from their path spend their life pursuing and exploring through conventional means, for example organised religion, a life of service dedicated to others, or meditation. There are many avenues and means of exploration of spirituality, including that through knowledge and wisdom. Whatever the means, the end product is the same. Sometimes the spiritual neglect in conventional health care is because it is not deemed scientific enough. It does not lend itself to easy measurement and only becomes important in health care when there is no hope of a cure.

The combination of faith, love, hope, compassion, truth, humility and justice forms important ingredients for a return to wholeness, despite our physical imperfections resulting from neglect, illness or disease. It is our inner strength of connection of soul and spirit that enables us to cope with our outer insecurities.[13]

> Heaven is the experience of sharing the joy, the peace and the love of God to the fullness of human capacity.
>
> *Father Laurence Freeman*[14]

References

1 Trungpa C. *Shambhala: The Sacred Path of the Warrior*. New York; Bantam Books; 1986.
2 Vickers A and Zollman C. ABC of complementary medicine, unconventional approach to nutritional medicine. *BMJ* 1999; 319:1419–22.
3 Zollman C and Vickers A. Users and practitioners of complementary medicine. *BMJ* 1999: 319: 836–8.
4 Lau CS, Morley KD and Belch JJ. Effects of fish oil supplementation on non-steroidal anti-inflammatory drug requirement in patients with mild rheumatoid arthritis – a double-blind placebo controlled study. *Br J Rheumatol* 1993; 32: 982–9.
5 Davies S and Stewart A. *Nutritional Medicine*. London: Pan; 1987.
6 O'Donohue J. *Anam Cara. Spiritual Wisdom from the Celtic World*. London: Bantam Press; 1999.
7 Fletcher GF, Baldy G, Steven NB *et al.*, American Heart Association. *Circulation* 1996; 94: 857–62.
8 Haslam D. What's new – tackling childhood obesity symposium – paediatric medicine. *Practitioner* 206; 250: 26–355.
9 Aldridge D. The therapeutic effects of music. In: Jonas WB and Crawford CC (eds). *Healing Intention and Energy Medicine*. London: Churchill Livingstone; 2003.
10 Halpern S and Savary L. *The Music and Sounds that Make us Whole*. San Francisco: Harper and Row; 1985.
11 Gerber R. *Vibrational Medicine*. Santa Fe: Bear and Co; 1988.
12 Sheldon MG. Spirituality healing and medicine. *Br J Gen Pract* 1992; 42: 38.
13 Judith A. *Eastern Body, Western Mind*. Berkeley, CA: Celestial Arts; 1996.
14 Dalai Lama. *The Good Heart*. London: Rider; 1997.

Further reading

- Brostoff J and Gamlin L. *Complete Guide to Food Allergy and Intolerance*. London: Bloomsbury; 1992.
- Conlin PR, Chow D, Miller ER *et al.* The effect of dietary patterns on blood pressure control in hypertensive patients: results from the Dietary Approaches to Stop Hypertension (DASH) trial. *Am J Hypertens* 2000; 13: 949–55.
- Dethlefsen T. *The Healing Power of Illness*. London: HarperCollins; 1997.
- Pizzorno MJ. *Encyclopaedia of Natural Medicine* (2e). London: Little Brown; 1999.
- Shapiro D. *Your Body Speaks Your Mind*. London: Piatkus; 1996.

Contacts

- *The Association of Professional Music Therapists*: www.apmt.org/; The Meadow, 68 Pierce Lane, Fulham, Cambridgeshire CB1 5DL
- *British Association of Nutritional Therapists*: 27 Old Gloucester Street, London WC1N 3XX; tel: 0870 606 1284
- *British Society for Allergy, Environmental and Nutritional Medicine (BSAENM) (Publications)*: PO Box 28, Totton, Southampton SO40 2ZA; tel. 01703 81 2124
- *The British Society for Music Therapy*: www.bsmt.org; 69 Avondale Avene, East Barnet, Herts EN4 8NB
- *Society for Promotion of Nutritional Therapy*: PO Box 47, Heathfield, East Sussex TN21 8ZX; tel: 01435 86 7007

Physical disease

23

Chronic disease

When meditating over a disease, I never think of finding a remedy for it, but instead, a means of preventing it.

Louis Pasteur (1822–1895)

In primary care, the majority of consultations are for chronic disease. The Quality Outcomes Framework (QOF), introduced in 2003 in the new General Medical Services (GMS) contract for primary care in the UK, is a significant advance. This ensures that regular surveillance and review is undertaken to monitor and treat a number of defined common chronic illnesses and disease.

Chronic disease management

The NHS in Britain provides a golden opportunity for continuity of care. This seamless health care can provide not only ongoing management of chronic disease but also a continuity of care where prevention of disease plays a major role. Lifestyle advice, screening and detection of common diseases can lead to early intervention, treatment and management.[1] In this way, fewer complications may arise, by controlling the disease process early and reducing morbidity and mortality.

The QOF model provides the opportunity to screen the population in each practice, with minimum standards and protocols laid down. The payment system in primary care in Britain ensures that the work is done before payment is made to a practice. The criteria in the QOF are reviewed regularly and adapted accordingly to meet the health needs of the population.

Integrated medicine can contribute to the quality of patient care and prevention. Before the QOF was established, chronic disease management was less uniform. Implementation of the QOF now enables national trends to be measured in the whole population, thus aiding chronic disease surveillance, prevention and management.

Having protocols for chronic disease management is a significant part of primary care. Where possible and practicable, patients can be taught to manage their disease. This type of management and support by patient, doctor, nurse, dietician and other healthcare professionals, as part of a team, puts the patients at the central core. Whatever the disease – asthma, diabetes, coronary heart disease, epilepsy and so forth – this empowers patients to self-regulate their own illness or disease. Without patient co-operation, education, interest and compliance, it is very difficult to achieve optimum management of a disease on behalf of the patient.[2] Therefore, integrated care does involve patient participation, and together with a holistic approach embraces a combination of factors leading to a successful management outcome in the longer term.

In the 1980s and 1990s, primary care led the thinking, planning and development of clinical audit and proactive care in chronic disease. Systematic and opportunistic screening combined will maximise early detection of chronic disease.[3]

Complementary care places the emphasis on the person, first and foremost. We illustrate the scope and diversity of complementary therapy and treatments with a selection of chronic diseases. The 'one size fits' all approach of conventional medicine is a recognised problem. Holistic care takes account of more than just the disease, it recognises the person as an individual and takes this into account in assessing, planning and long-term management.

The following chronic conditions have been chosen to illustrate the place of complementary therapies in their management. For additional information on each therapy refer to the appropriate chapter.

Irritable bowel syndrome

Dietary changes can have a dramatic effect on irritable bowel syndrome (IBS): a low-fibre diet often has a beneficial effect (*see* Chapter 22). This common condition is suitable for complementary treatment once the diagnosis is confirmed:

Herbal medicine

Camomile, peppermint and ginger infusions are used to help calm the bowel and relieve pain.

Homeopathy

- *Argentum nitricum*: this is used for colicky abdominal pain, with flatulence, anticipatory anxiety and where the patient has a preference for sweet food.
- *Colocynth*: this remedy is indicated in griping abdominal pains that are better for bending over and doubling up or for applying pressure and warmth on the abdomen.

Hypnotherapy

Several studies have shown hypnotherapy to be effective in the treatment of severe IBS. A high response rate has been shown in the investigation of mechanisms and effects of symptoms.[4,5]

Inflammatory bowel disease (Crohn's disease and ulcerative colitis)

Acupunture

The gallbladder, liver and stomach meridians are stimulated for pain relief (*see* Chapter 7).

Herbal medicine

Slippery elm used twice daily is beneficial to alleviate symptoms.

Homeopathy

- *Natrum sulphuricum*: this remedy is used to alleviate colic and flatulence.
- *The constitutional remedy* is often also required (*see* Chapter 12).

Haemorrhoids

Aromatherapy

Application of essential oils of camomile, frankincense, myrrh, cypress or pepper-mint can be used by putting them in bath water.

Herbal medicine

Witch hazel, comfrey or horse chestnuts ointment can be applied locally.

Homeopathy

- *Aesculus*: for stabbing, tearing pains associated with constipation
- *Aloe*: indicated in prolapsed grape-like haemorrhoids
- *Hamamelis*: helps in soreness and bruising
- *Nitric acid*: relieves the burning pain associated with anal fissure
- *Nux vomica*: in irritable, chilly individuals who are always in a hurry
- *Pulsatilla*: for thirstless, gentle, fair-haired individuals, usually female
- *Sulphur*: used in patients who are always warm with a red peri-anal area and who have a tendency towards either constipation or diarrhoea

Osteoarthritis and rheumatoid arthritis

Acupuncture

In a follow-up study over one year, 93% (13 out of 14) patients responded to acupuncture treatment for metatarsalgia. The effect was reported to be long-lasting. Only two patients had a relapse during the study period.[6]

Homeopathy

- *Bryonia*: for pain that is worse in damp weather and on movement
- *Rhus toxicodendron*: for stiffness in the joints on waking, improving on movement
- *Rhododendron*: for pain that is worse in damp weather

Herbal medicine (for osteoarthritis)

Glucosamine and chondroitin are effective in this condition. A 3-year randomised controlled study of 212 patients compared glucosamine with placebo. This showed that in patients over 50 years of age on 1500 mg oral glucosamine sulphate daily, compared to placebo, there were significant benefits. The average joint space was 5.44 mm at baseline. With placebo there was a mean narrowing of 0.33 mm over the 3 years. With glucosamine there was no narrowing. There was a significant reduction in pain for 20–25% of patients.[7]

Case study 23.1

Fiona, a 52-year-old nurse, was diagnosed with rheumatoid arthritis 9 years previously. She presented with generalised arthralgia of the large joints. Her rheumatoid factor was positive with sheep cell agglutination titre (SCAT) of 1 in 80, which then increased to 1 in 40 three months later. The joints were mildly swollen and the erythrocyte sedimentation rate (ESR) was 36 mm/h. She had morning stiffness, which improved after mobilising. Rhus toxico-dendron, a homeopathic remedy, was prescribed on a weekly basis. She reported a marked improvement. The haemoglobin was normal initially, but later she developed a mild anaemia that was normocytic and normochronic, and her serum ferritin was low. She was treated with an oral iron preparation. Rhus toxicodendron was prescribed every few months whenever her joints became inflamed.

   Five years previously, at the age of 47 years she had become perimeno-pausal, her luteinising hormone (LH) and follicle stimulating hormone (FSH) were elevated. She was prescribed homeopathic Sepia and Belladonna for the hot flushes. Three months later she was given Sulphur as a constitutional homeopathic remedy. Her rheumatoid factor remained positive with a SCAT of 1 in 40.

   She improved markedly over the following 4 years, and her rheumatoid factor reverted to negative; this was repeated a year later and it remained negative. Her condition clinically was much improved.

Backache

Acupuncture

Acupuncture is particularly useful when physiotherapy and other forms of treatment are too painful to apply. If there is muscle spasm and tension, acupuncture treatment can relieve this to allow other forms of manipulation treatments to be used.

Alexander technique

Musicians are routinely taught this technique for prevention of neck, back and spinal problems during performance. This can also be used to alleviate spinal problems (*see* Chapter 16).

Chiropractic

For mechanical causes of backache, the chiropractor will apply gentle but precise pressure and gentle massage manipulation to restore normal function to the joints.

Herbal remedies

Willow bark and Devil's claw are commonly used in treating backache. Herbal remedies should be considered 'the first course of action' a Cochrane review concludes.[8]

Homeopathy

- *Arnica*: where injury is present
- *Bryonia*: for continuous pain
- *Ruta*: for continuous ligament pain
- *Rhus toxicodendron*: the pain improves on movement initially
- *Magnesia phosphorica*: this is useful in sciatica

Osteopathy

After a full diagnostic work-up, a registered osteopath will apply manipulation to the spine by pressing, pulling and twisting gently. For prolapsed intervertebral discs or chronic degenerative problems, several treatment sessions may be required.

Reflexology

Reflex zones corresponding to the area of the spine are massaged and stimulated.

Osteoporosis

A balanced diet with adequate intake of **calcium** and **regular exercise** are essential for the treatment and prevention of osteoporosis.

Therapies that can be used as part of a prevention programme are:

- *yoga* (*see* Chapter 21)
- *homeopathy*: the constitutional remedy may help slow the process down (*see* Chapter 12).

It is important that conventional bisphosphonate medication is considered if a significant degree of osteoporosis is present.

Leg cramps

Massage

Gently rubbing the affected area can produce relief.

Herbal medicine

Crampbark and ginger infusions are often effective.

Aromatherapy

A mixture of lemon grass, marjoram and basil in a bath or rub can be used.

Homeopathy

Cuprum metallicum, Nux vomica, Calcarea carbonica and Arnica montana are helpful, depending on the homeopathic history.

Myalgic encephalomyelitis (ME; post-viral syndrome)

Acupuncture

For relief of symptoms without side effects. *See* Chapter 7.

Aromatherapy

- Lavender helps induce relaxation to alleviate fatigue.
- Oil of lemon calms the mind.

Herbal medicine

St John's wort, wild oats and vervain are all used to induce relaxation.

Homeopathy

A constitutional remedy is prescribed on the cluster of symptoms of an individual patient (*see* Chapter 12).[9]

Cerebrovascular accident

Patients with a cerebrovascular accident (CVA) or transient ischaemic attack (TIA) will need urgent investigation and long-term rehabilitation.

Complementary therapies are used for symptomatic relief and rehabilitation: massage/physiotherapy, speech therapy, aromatherapy and treatments that generally produce a relaxation effect.

Neuralgias

Acupuncture

Appropriate points are manipulated daily initially and repeated when the pain is acute.

Aromatherapy

Facial neuralgia can also be treated with clove oil, basil and eucalyptus used as a lotion.

Homeopathy

- *Arsenicum album*: for burning pains in a restless person
- *Colocynth*: for tearing pain made worse by cold, relieved by pressure
- *Kalmia*: used for right-sided neuralgia
- *Spigelia*: for left-sided tearing, facial pain which can be made worse by pressure

Multiple sclerosis

There is often significant stress and depression in patients with multiple sclerosis (MS). Most therapies associated with stress management are helpful in this condition:

- aromatherapy
- massage
- Reiki
- reflexology
- yoga.

The physical and emotional symptoms of MS can be alleviated by the expert use of homeopathic remedies. Associated stress can be relieved by the holistic approach.[10]

Homeopathy

- *Agaricus*: used to help sharp, shooting pains
- *Causticum*: used to control incontinence of urine
- *Hypericum*: for tingling sensations and nerve pains
- *Kali phosphoricum*: for fatigue and pain with back and limb pains made worse by exercise
- *Magnesia phosphorica*: relieves spasms and jerking of the limbs
- *Natrum muriaticum*: for depression that often accompanies MS
- The homeopathic constitutional remedy may help generally (*see* Chapter 12)

Case study 23.2

Anne, a single 43 year old, with a 7-year history of MS, was housebound, overweight, depressed, exhausted and had not been able to work for over a year. She also had problems with muscle spasms and cramps. She lived alone with little help and felt trapped in her own body.

Her integrated management was as follows:

- *homeopathy*: Natrum muriaticum and Calcarea carbonica for depression; Cannabis indica for the muscle spasms
- *Reiki*: this had a relaxing effect on the whole system and reduced the spasms; one-hour energy healing sessions each week for 8 weeks were given
- *diet and supplements*: a healthy balanced diet was essential for her optimum health; calcium, magnesium and zinc supplements were taken daily
- *exercise*: Anne started swimming regularly, just 4 weeks after her initial treatment with Reiki and homeopathy
- *mobility*: her own mobility improved and she was able to get around more easily, though still relying on crutches. She also developed enough confidence to buy a motorised scooter, which enabled her to return to part-time work.

This lady illustrates well the integration of complementary therapies and conventional care and the successful outcome accomplished. Her dignity, self-respect and self-help have given her a different perspective on life.

Thyroid disorders

Homeopathy

Thyroxine (homeopathic remedy) can be used in hypothyroidism where the thyroid-stimulating hormone (TSH) is monitored regularly. If, however, the TSH increases to 10 mu/l or more and homeopathic treatment does not control the disease adequately, then conventional treatment should be on stand by. In thyrotoxicosis, however, conventional medicines should be used, as a first-line management. Homeopathic remedies can be used subsequently for symptomatic relief.

Case study 23.3

Sandra, a 69 year old, presented with a 5-year history of hypothyroidism. For the first 8 months, she tolerated conventional 25 μg of thyroxine. As the dose was subsequently increased to 75 μg, she developed palpitations, which made her feel unwell. An ambulatory ECG showed a sinus tachycardia. She was therefore changed to eltroxin and as the dose was increased she collapsed. Six months prior to seeking homeopathic treatment she stopped her conventional medication altogether. At the beginning of treatment, a free thyroxine

(T_4) was 11 mmol/l and TSH 14.6 u/l. She reported falling asleep easily. Homeopathic thyroxine 6c potency twice daily was prescribed long term.

Her thyroid function tests (TFTs) were monitored regularly. Homeopathic thyroxine was eventually increased to 200 c potency once a week. Six months after commencing the higher potency her TSH was 6.4 mu/l and T_4 12 mmol/l. Her hypothyroidism is now under control and she is quite stable.

Her condition improved markedly and her weight remained steady. Her TFTs were monitored regularly to ensure her stability and also provided evidence of the efficacy of homeopathy.

Macular degeneration

The Age-Related Eye Disease Study suggests that in patients with the unilateral advanced age-related macular degeneration, a specific combination of high doses of zinc, anti-oxidant and vitamins helps prevent advanced disease and visual acuity deterioration in the unaffected eye.[11] This applies only to non-smokers; it does not seem to help smokers or ex-smokers.

Advice should be given on smoking cessation and eating a healthy balanced diet rich in green vegetables.

Diabetes mellitus

Regular monitoring of diabetes is always useful for long-term prevention of complications. Complementary therapies are used to stabilise and improve the general mental and physical health of a patient and also help add to the quality of life. For diabetics whose condition is controlled by diet alone, therapies can also be used to maintain a good health balance and effective control. It is important that a dietician is involved with the care of all diabetic patients.

During stressful and difficult times the following complementary therapies can be used to indirectly influence blood sugar control and create balance:

- aromatherapy
- reflexology
- massage
- homeopathy
- Reiki
- yoga.

For their general health, many patients with diabetes mellitus use complementary therapies.[12]

The following homeopathic remedies can be considered:

- *Argentum nitricum*: used to control anticipatory anxiety
- *Natrum muriaticum*: useful when depression is a feature
- *Phosphoric acid*: indicated in nervous exhaustion
- *Silicea*: in thin, chilly, sweating individuals with loss of stamina.

Cardiology

Before embarking on treatment, conventional or complementary, it is paramount to have an accurate diagnosis. This needs thorough history taking alongside an examination and subsequent investigation. The patient then can benefit from the safest and most appropriate management plan. The following case study with a cardiologist and homeopath providing joint care illustrates this well.

Case study 23.4: palpitations managed by homeopathic treatment

Edward, a 64-year-old retired lecturer, presented with intermittent palpitations over the past 10 years. Initially he was investigated by a cardiologist; this included a 24-hour ECG, which was normal.

He was thin, very concise in giving his history and was a very tidy person to the point of fastidiousness. There was a family history of heart disease; his mother died aged 47 years from an acute myocardial infarction. He smoked seven cigarettes a day. His TFTs, full blood count, biochemistry and cholesterol were within normal range. He was normotensive with a regular pulse of 72 beats/minute.

Homeopathic Arsenicum was prescribed, which settled his palpitations within a few days. He presented a year later with a recurrence of the palpitations and again treated with Arsenicum. At this point however, he was referred for a further cardiological assessment to ensure that there was no underlying cause. He underwent an exercise ECG and a heart scan, both of which were reported as normal. The cardiologist reported that 'the palpitations had been due to episodic premature activity without any obvious substrate in terms of underlying heart disease.' A repeat of Arsenicum resolved his palpitations and he continues to remain well.

Asthma

Asthma in children and adults involves an allergic element with house dust mite, pollens or feathers. Stress and anxiety may also be contributory factors. Atopic individuals have eczema with the asthma. A holistic approach by a homeopathic physician will treat the skin and the asthma as part of the individual and not as separate diseases. In Britain, 15% of children are affected with asthma.

Acupuncture

Meridians on the ear lobe are stimulated with effective relief of asthma.

Aromatherapy

Eucalyptus, juniper, wintergreen, peppermint and rosemary oils are applied to the chest at night. These can also be inhaled from a tissue when dyspnoea is present.

Herbal medicine

The Pasque flower herb relieves tension and improves relaxation. Thyme and euphorbia infusions relax muscles and loosen phlegm.

Homeopathy

- *Arsenicum album*: for thirsty, anxious individuals who feel better sitting up and are restless and chilly
- *Antimonium tartaricum*: for cold, clammy patients, suffering from exhaustion and 'noisy' breathing
- *Ipecacuanha*: for patients where the chest feels as if it has a heavy weight, accompanied with nausea and vomiting
- *Kali carb*: for chilly, pale, tired patients, whose asthma is worse between 2 and 4 pm
- *Natrum sulphuricum*: for asthma associated with early morning diarrhoea, also for cases where the asthma is worse in damp weather

Massage

Gentle massage when breathing is difficult allows postural drainage for any mucus. The patient lies face down with the head lower than the chest and this can also help calm and relax the system.

Reflexology

The areas of the feet relating to the lungs are massaged primarily, and this helps relieve difficult breathing.

Essential hypertension

A reduction in dietary salt is always advisable. Exercise (once the hypertension is under control), reducing stress and maintaining weight control are also important factors. A woman on the combined oral contraceptive pill or hormone replacement therapy should discontinue this medication, as oestrogen can contribute to increased blood pressure. Alcohol and coffee intake should also be reduced.

Therapies alone may control mild hypertension. In some cases it may well be necessary to add smaller doses of conventional drugs to maintain long-term control.

Acupuncture

Various meridians in the body are used to treat essential hypertension with good effect.[13]

Aromatherapy

Lavender oil in the bath or as a massage will help calm the system and relieve stress.

Homeopathy

- *Argentum nitricum*: useful in anticipatory anxiety
- *Crataegus tincture*: a specific remedy for essential hypertension
- *Sulphur*: useful for hypertension in the menopause

In addition to the remedies listed above, the constitutional remedy (*see* Chapter 12, p. 71) may also be indicated.

Case study 23.5

Andrea is a 72-year-old retired professional with essential hypertension and blood pressure (BP) readings in the region of 168/100 mmHg. In her first homeopathic assessment her BP was 180/110 mmHg sitting. After 5 minutes of meditation, this was reduced to 170/100 mmHg. She was prescribed homeopathic Crataegus tincture (concentrated Hawthorn berries) to be taken 5 drops twice daily. Three years later her BP remained within normal range in the region of 135/80 mmHg, with a normal heart rate.

Epilepsy

Relaxation can help control petit mal or grand mal epilepsy. The main therapies indicated for relaxation are:

- aromatherapy
- reflexology
- yoga
- Reiki
- homeopathy
- meditation.

Benign prostatic hypertrophy

It is important to obtain a full history in benign prostatic hypertrophy (BPH), conduct a detailed examination including rectal examination and investigate to exclude malignancy.

Herbal medicine

Saw palmetto (*see* Chapter 11).

Homeopathy

- *Sabal serulata*: this remedy is beneficial when nocturia with perineal pain is a feature
- *Clematis erecta*: used for intermittent urinary flow
- *Equisetum*: indicated mainly for terminal dysuria

- *Staphysagria*: used in recurrent urinary tract infections
- *Causticum*: used in stress incontinence, particularly in the elderly

Coronary heart disease

The role of complementary therapies in coronary heart disease (CHD) is primarily in prevention.[14]

Whether the body is under stress in established CHD or for prevention, reducing the risk factor associated with this condition is paramount.[1]

Important factors in coronary heart disease

- *Family history*
- *Sex*: CHD is more common in males
- *Hypertension* increases risk of CHD and stroke
- *Lifestyle* (*see* Chapter 22): there is no substitute for a healthy lifestyle
- *Stress* (*see* Chapter 3)
- *Obesity*
- *Exercise*: a sedentary lifestyle predisposes to CHD. One half hour session five times weekly is recommended in prevention
- *Smoking*
- *Alcohol*:
    2 units a day on average reduces incidence of CHD
    – long term, excessive intake increases the risk
- *Cholesterol/lipid profile*: diet alone can reduce total cholesterol by up to 30%. The statin group of drugs can reduce the level further
- *Diet*: excessive salt in food increases the risk of CHD and strokes. The Food Standards Agency (FSA) has recommended a significant reduction in salt in food to reduce the risk in the general population.[15] Also a high-fibre diet is recommended with the addition of fish oil.

> *A wise man should consider that health is the greatest of human blessings, and learn how by his own thoughts to derive benefit from his illness.*
>
> *Hippocrates*

References

1 Demetriou A. Preventative medicine and health promotion. In: Fry J and Bouchier-Hayes T (eds). *The Medical Annual*. Bristol: Clinical Press; 1991. pp. 119–28.
2 *From Ideas to Action: improving chronic disease management*. Department of Health Conference; 2004 18 May, London UK. www.dh.gov.uk (accessed 13 October 2006).
3 Demetriou A. SOS, Systematic Opportunistic Screening, practising practical prevention. *Manchester Med* 1986; 2: 9.
4 Whorwell PJ, Prior A and Colgan SM. Hypnotherapy in severe-irritable-bowel-syndrome – further experience. *Gut* 1987; 28: 423–5.
5 Whorwell PJ. Review article: the history of hypnotherapy and its role in the irritable bowel syndrome. *Aliment Pharmacol Ther* 2005; 22: 1061–7.
6 Stellon A. Metatarsalgia: treatment by acupuncture. *Acupunct Med* 1977; 15: 17–18.

7 Reginster JY, Deroisy R and Rovati LC. Long term effects of glucosamine sulphate on osteo-arthritis progression: a randomised placebo-controlled trial. *Lancet* 2001; 357: 251–6.

8 Cagnier JJ, van Tulder M, Berman B *et al*. Herbal medicine for low back pain (Cochrane Review). *The Cochrane Library, Issue 2*. Oxford: Update Software; 2006.

9 Jenkins M. Thoughts on the management of myalgic encephalomyelitis. *Br Homeopath J* 1989; 78: 6–14.

10 Apel A, Greim B and Zettl UK. How frequently do patients with multiple sclerosis use complementary and alternative medicine? *Complement Ther Med* 2005; 13: 258–63.

11 Anon. Nutritional supplements for macular degeneration. *Drug Ther Bull* 2006; 44: 9–11.

12 Yeh GY, Eisenberg DM, Davis RB *et al*. Use of complementary and alternative medicine among persons with diabetes mellitus: results of a national survey. *Am J Public Health* 2002; 92: 1648–52.

13 Longhurst JC. Hypertension: acupuncture found to lower elevations in blood pressure. *Proceedings of The Medical Devices and Surgical Technology Week*. 24 April 2005; Atlanta, USA, p.233.

14 Patel C, Marmot MG, Terry DJ *et al*. Trial of relaxation in reducing coronary risk: four year follow up. *BMJ* 1985; 29: 1103–6.

15 Corruzi P, Parati G, Brambilla L *et al*. Effects of salt sensitivity on neural cardiovascular regulation in essential hypertension. *Hypertension* 2005; 46: 1321–6.

Further reading

- Demetriou A and Coyle M. Complementary medicine. In: Shukla RB and Brooks D (eds). *A Guide to Care of the Elderly*. London: HMSO; 1996. pp. 339–48.

- Spence DS and Thompson EA. Homeopathic treatment for chronic disease: a 6-year, university-hospital outpatient observational study. *J Altern Complement Med* 2005; 11: 793–8.

- Walker AF, Marakis G, Simpson E *et al*. Hypotensive effects of hawthorn for patients with diabetes taking prescription drugs: a randomised controlled trial. *Br J Gen Pract* 2006; 56: 437–43.

24

Dermatology

There is security and rest in the wisdom of the eternal scripture.

James 1:5

Skin conditions are generally distressing and recurrent, and often chronic, unsightly and painful. A holistic approach with a successful outcome can transform a patient's life. The commonest dermatological conditions in general practice are dealt with in this section. More details on the therapies discussed in each disease process are found in the relevant chapters.

Urticaria

There are many causes of urticaria:

- physical
- emotional stress
- food allergies, especially those containing salicylates or food additives, colourings such as tartarazine, or foods such as strawberries and shellfish
- drugs, notably aspirin
- fungal infections
- nettle stings
- jellyfish, insects and contact with furry animals.

The cause of urticaria can often be identified from a detailed history. An exclusion diet may also be appropriate to highlight the offending additive. For symptomatic relief, as an alternative to antihistamines, the following therapies can be considered.

Homeopathy

- *Urtica urens*: this is a common remedy used to relieve acute symptoms of stings from nettles and other plants
- *Apis*: for oedema of the eyelids and lips
- *Natrum muriaticum*: indicated in chronic, recurrent urticara often made worse by stress and exercise
- *Rhus toxicodendron*: helps relieve burning and itchy rashes
- *Sulphur*: for red, itchy rashes made worse by heat. The patient is often constitutionally warm
- *Arsenicum*: given for urticaria in patients with restlessness and anxiety

Herbal medicine

A cool infusion of camomile or chickweed to alleviate itching may be used (*see* Chapters 11 and 20).

Acne

In teenagers especially, acne can be a very distressing problem. They are a very self-conscious group of patients and worry about their appearance. Instead of oral antibiotics many patients prefer a more natural approach.

Herbal medicine

Antibacterial and anti-inflammatory skin washes can be applied. Calendula, camomile and yarrow elder or lavender can be used to make up herbal applications. Internal remedies include burdock, echinacea and red clover. These are thought to cleanse the body and help reduce spots and any recurrence.

Aromatherapy

The skin affected is bathed regularly with distilled water in which lavender, juniper and cajuput essential oils are added.

Tea-tree oil applied to the spots can deal with any infection.

Nutritional medicine

Avoiding kelp and tonics rich in iodine can often minimise aggravation of the acne. Treatment with zinc can also be effective. A healthy, balanced diet is essential to maintain good healthy skin (*see* Chapter 22).

Homeopathy

- *Sulphur*: for warm, dry skin, in acne of long standing
- *Calcarea sulphurica*: for weeping, pustules with yellow crusts
- *Hepar sulphuris*: for the presence of pustules with boils
- *Kali bromatum*: for itchy spots causing restless sleep in a fidgety individual
- *Pulsatilla*: used in fair-haired females, who weep easily and dislike a stuffy atmosphere
- *Antimonium tartaricum*: used where pustules predominate
- *Silicea*: used for patients where the skin scars easily
- *Sepia*: used for patients with a low mood, where premenstrual exacerbation of the acne and low energy are the main features

Case study 24.1

Diane, a 14 year old, had quite severe pustular acne. She was low in mood and had little energy. A chilly person by nature, self-conscious and despondent, her acne was often worse premenstrually. She was not thirsty and could only take small meals, feeling full easily. She was irritable premenstrually and pale in complexion with greasy hair. Her posture displayed all the hallmarks of low self-esteem. Homeopathically, her constitutional remedy, Sepia was given, mid-cycle. On review two months later, her skin returned to normal, the acne had resolved fully, she became brighter, happier and more confident. Improvement was sustained long term, a truly dramatic response, physically and emotionally.

Viral warts

Children and parents alike are keen to cure unsightly warts, particularly on the fingers and face. As an alternative to cryotherapy the following therapies can be used.

Acupuncture

Treatment is focused on meridian points around the warts and also on the lung and large intestine areas. It is thought that these acupuncture points stimulate anti-inflammatory defences and produce an immune system support with good effect.

Hypnotherapy

Under hypnosis, the patient is given suggestions that the warts will fade away eventually and drop off.

Homeopathy

- *Thuja*: for cauliflower-type warts, and is also the most frequently used remedy in treating warts
- *Causticum*: for warts on the face, eyelids and fingertips, and for painful verrucas
- *Nitric acid*: indicated for warts that itch or sting
- *Natrum carbonicum*: for ulcerated warts
- *Dulcamara*: used where there are fleshy warts, particularly on the dorsum of hands
- *Antimonium crudum*: a remedy specifically for horny warts
- *Calcarea*: used in multiple small, itchy, stinging warts, which discharge or bleed
- *Kali muriaticum*: this is the main remedy for warts on the hands
- *Sepia*: often used for large, dark warts

The remedies are given for several weeks on a weekly basis, until the warts resolve. Many homeopaths give two remedies, one to be taken midweek and the other at weekends, over 8 weeks. This depends on the appearance and the length of time the warts have been present.

Eczema

This chronic skin disease is often accompanied by asthma, and this combination is known as atopy. As much distress is often caused by the topical creams and ointments as by the disease itself. Complementary therapies, particularly homeopathy, help considerably in controlling this condition.

Acupuncture

Meridians are treated that correspond to the stomach, spleen, lungs and large intestine. If the practitioner assesses that the liver is 'not functioning properly' and contributing to the eczema, then dietary advice is suggested, for example alcohol, coffee, dairy products and fatty food are best avoided.

Aromatherapy

Essential oils that are commonly used include camomile, geranium, hyssop, sandalwood, juniper and lavender. For dryness, calendula oil is often indicated.

Homeopathy

- *Sulphur*: for erythematous, dry, itchy skin aggravated by heat
- *Graphites*: for the presence of a yellow discharge, especially from behind the ears
- *Petroleum*: this is a remedy used when the skin cracks easily
- *Rhus toxicodendron*: for itchy vesicles that are worse at night. The eczema is worse in damp weather and improves by keeping warm
- *Hepar sulphuris*: for infected eczema that is worse in cold weather
- *Arsenicum album*: indicated in dry, burning skin, which is aggravated by the cold

Chinese herbal remedies

Chinese herbs are widely used, are tailored to the individual needs and should only be prescribed by a **registered herbalist**. The side-effect of herbs used for atopic eczema is hepatoxicity, which can range from mild liver enzyme alterations to chronic liver failure. Germander (Teucrum chamaedrys) may cause hepatitis and even cirrhosis of the liver. Chaparral has also been known to cause similar problems.[1-3]

Case study 24.2: infantile eczema

Joseph, an 8-month-old boy, presented with a 2-month history of eczema and asthma (atopy). He weighed 4.2 kg at birth, had normal developmental milestones, was bottle fed with cow's milk and had a placid nature with a tendency to 'head sweating'. He was treated homeopathically with Calcarea carbonica granules and three days later his skin became itchy and more erythematous (in homeopathic theory this is known as 'an aggravation'). A week later the skin had improved significantly. Two weeks later he developed a viral upper respiratory tract infection and the eczema returned to its pretreatment state. The eczema had become infected, and antibiotics were prescribed. A week later the eczema had improved leaving a dry skin. A further dose of Calcarea was prescribed (6 weeks after the initial dose) with a marked improvement. The child remained well for 6 months until he developed chickenpox, which was then followed by dry skin in the nappy area and the flexures of his upper limbs. He had a tendency to constipation and was a warm child (bodily). Salbutamol syrup for his asthma was prescribed by his GP. At this stage he was given homeopathic Sulphur. Six weeks later he was much improved, alert, feeding well and his cough had resolved and the salbutamol was then discontinued.

He had no further problems with the atopy for over 10 years. He presented again at the age of 12 years with a 3-month history of recurrence of his eczema, on his face and wrists. A further dose of Sulphur was given. His eczema improved over the next few weeks.

This case study illustrates how infections can trigger chronic conditions and alter the status of the immune system, precipitating underlying disease. The response to homeopathic remedies in this child was successful, illustrating the benefits of integrated medicine.

Psoriasis

This can be a difficult condition to treat whether by conventional or complementary medicine. The following therapies may be considered.

Herbal medicine

Infusion of dandelion root, burdock and red clover flowers may help (*see* Chapters 11 and 20).

Homeopathy

- *Sulphur*: used where there are erythematous, itchy plaques present
- *Graphites*: used when patients display a yellow discharge especially behind the ears
- *Petroleum*: used where the main feature is dry cracked skin, which is worse in winter
- *Arsenicum album*: used for symptoms of burning skin, in a restless, chilly, thirsty person
- *Kali arsenicosum*: indicated when the skin displays scaly areas, which are aggravated by warmth

Aromatherapy

- *Sandalwood oil* for dry scaly patches displayed anywhere on the body
- *Bergamot and lavender oils* keep the condition under control, and can also be applied as a lotion or oil and added to the bath water

Leg ulcers

Leg ulcers are distressing and often become chronic, needing much expert nursing attention and frequent dressings. The following therapies have been widely used.

Herbal medicine

Manuka honey is applied topically to ulcerated areas over a period of time.[4]

Homeopathy

Mercurius is just one example of a remedy that can be used to good effect. It is given orally over a number of weeks and dressings applied in the usual way. A constitutional remedy is often used in addition (*see* Chapter 12, p. 71).

Magnetism therapy

Magnetic leg wraps called '4 Ulcer Care' have been evaluated as being therapeutic and a cost-effective treatment that saves on dressings and nurse time.[5]

> *Happiness is a product of the mind, of attitude and thought. It comes from you, not to you. To be happy you must choose to be happy: the scripture says, 'as a man thinks in his heart, so is he'.*
>
> Proverbs 23:7

References

1 Department of Immunology, UCL Medical School. London UK. Association of immunology changes with clinical efficacy in atopic eczema patients treated with traditional Chinese herbal therapy (Zenaphyte). *Int Arch Allergy Immunol* 1996; 109: 243–9.
2 Kirbv A and Schmidt R. The antioxidant activity of Chinese herbs for eczema and of placebo herbs. *J Ethnopharmacol* 1997; 56: 103–8.
3 Sheehan MP and Atherton DJ. A controlled trial of traditional Chinese medicinal plants in widespread non-exudative atopic eczema. *Br J Dermatol* 1992; 126: 179–84.
4 Greenwood D. Honey for superficial wounds and ulcers. *Lancet* 1993; 341: 90–1.
5 Eccles NK and Hollinworth BA. A pilot study to determine whether a static magnetic device can promote chronic leg ulcer healing. *J Wound Care* 2005; 14: 64.

Further reading

- Smith SA, Baker AE and Williams JH. Effective treatment of seborrhoeic dermatitis using a low dose, oral homeopathic medication consisting of potassium bromide, sodium bromide, nickel sulphate and sodium chloride in a double-blind, placebo-controlled study. *Altern Med Rev* 2002; 7: 59–67.

25

Ear, nose and throat

Silence at the proper season is wisdom, and better than any speech.

Plutarch

The most common and acute conditions are discussed in relation to an integrated approach in treatment. Many of these diseases are distressing and amenable to complementary therapy/integrated care. For further details on each therapy, see relevant chapters.

Benign paroxysmal positional vertigo

When a complementary therapy relieves vertigo, it usually does so without the need for long-term medication. When there is a recurrence, then a repeat of the therapy may be all that is needed.

Acupuncture

The gallbladder and kidney meridians are stimulated and used in the treatment of vertigo.

Homeopathy

- *Cocculus*: for ongoing dizziness, regardless of position
- *Conium*: used when vertigo is worse on turning the head or in the supine position
- *Belladonna*: where otitis media is present, causing dizziness
- *Bryonia*: for dizziness brought on by eye movements
- *Borax*: for when symptoms become worse by looking down
- *Natrum muriaticum*: where headaches are present

The Epley manoeuvre (particle repositioning)

The theory is that benign paroxysmal positional vertigo is caused by otoconial debris in the posterior semi-circular canal of the ear.[1] The Epley manoeuvre is a non-drug method of treatment carried out as follows:

- *stage 1*: the patient sits on the couch and is asked to turn their head to the side that you suspect is the affected ear. If this is not clear, guess the side initially. Ask the patient to recline, if the vertigo comes on then that is the correct side. If there is no vertigo, then ask the patient to turn the head the other way and to recline again
- *stage 2*: the patient now sits looking straight ahead, with eyes open turning the head 45 degrees to the affected side (say the left)

- *stage 3*: at the count of 3, the patient reclines past the horizontal position. The patient's head is caught by the doctor, so that the fall coincides with the head over the edge of the couch, this manoeuvre requires confidence on the patient's part. Dizziness will often be triggered during the fall. The head is turned to the right. Hold for 30 seconds
- *stage 4*: ask the patient to roll onto their right side – the head still turned to the right, hence facing the floor. Hold for 30 seconds
- *stage 5*: the patient then sits upright, still looking over their right shoulder. This may bring on more vertigo. Hold for 30 seconds
- *stage 6*: the head is then turned to the midline with the neck flexed, at 45 degrees. Hold for 30 seconds.

If the patient then reclines and there is now no dizziness, the treatment has been successful.

If there is a recurrence, the Epley manoeuvre can be repeated. Neurological causes should be considered if the manoeuvre is not effective.

Case study 25.1

Jack, a 34-year old male, presented with a 4-week history of dizziness. He had nystagmus on looking to the right. There were no other neurological signs. A 2-week course of betahistine had no effect what so ever. The Epley manoeuvre was performed, which resolved his vertigo instantly. The betahistine was discontinued. There were no further problems when he was seen a year later.

Travel sickness

The following therapies can be very effective in this distressing condition.

Acupressure

This is a simple manoeuvre and easy for anyone to use. Pressure is applied to a point about three fingers' width above the medial aspect of the wrist, which is pressed centrally with the middle finger. Wristbands are now widely available and perform the same function.

Aromatherapy

Ginger and peppermint essential oils on a tissue can be inhaled regularly during a journey to relieve the sickness.

Homeopathy

- *Aconite napellis*: this remedy is indicated in patients displaying a fear of death and impending disaster, which accompanies the travel sickness
- *Borax*: for fear of sudden, downward motion, in air travel
- *Cocculus*: for nausea, increased salivation, with dizziness and tiredness

- *Nux vomica*: for irritable individuals feeling cold, with an occipital headache
- *Petroleum*: in dizziness made worse by sitting up or on hearing a loud noise
- *Rhus toxicodendron*: for patients in whom the sickness feels better on lying down

Otitis media

Children are particularly vulnerable to the side-effects of conventional drugs (*see* Chapter 28).[2] The following therapies can be easily integrated.

Herbal medicine

Herbal remedies are available over the counter, for example cayenne willow bark or boneset herbal remedies, and they are used to treat the fever.

Homeopathy

- *Aconite napellis*: given initially for anxiety and restlessness soon after the onset of infection
- *Belladonna*: this remedy is given for fever, being flushed, and unusually sensitive to touch
- *Pulsatilla*: for an individual in pain who tends to weep easily

---

Case study 25.2

Derek, an 84-year-old retired professional male, developed a sore throat. On the second day of his illness he complained of intense right-sided earache. There was no evidence of a discharge. He had otitis media with an injected tympanic membrane and was prescribed Belladonna 30c potency at half hourly intervals for six doses, then at 4 hourly for the next 24 hours. The following day his symptoms had resolved completely.

Hay fever

In conventional treatment a patient may need eye drops, a nasal spray and oral antihistamines. In severe cases of hay fever, an intramuscular steroid injection may be indicated. Complementary treatments are much more acceptable and palatable to children. Prevention, by reducing exposure to pollen, will also help.

Acupuncture

Needles are inserted to stimulate the points of the large intestine governing the lung and spleen meridians.

Hypnotherapy

Hypnotherapy is helpful for symptomatic relief and in preventing further attacks.

Homeopathy

- *Arsenicum album*: the main features suitable for Arsenicum are burning of the throat and eyes, and rhinorrhoea is usually present. It is used in anxious individuals, whose symptoms are also improved by keeping warm
- *Gelsemium*: for sneezing, dizziness, lacrimation and restlessness
- *Allium cepa*: for a burning nasal discharge and a degree of photophobia
- *Euphrasia*: used in patients who have a thick burning discharge from the eyes and nose, a productive cough and whose symptoms are worse indoors
- *Sabadilla*: for burning, itchy eyes, photophobia, blocked nose and general irritability
- *Pulsatilla*: the symptoms for this remedy are yellow nasal and eye discharges, which are better in the open air
- *Sanguinaria*: for chronic rhinitis with dry and congested nasal membranes

Catarrh

This distressing symptom often follows a respiratory infection, particularly in people who smoke.

Aromatherapy

Some of the common remedies used are basil, eucalyptus, lavender, lemon, thyme or cedar wood oil in a bath or as steam inhalations.

Acupuncture

This treatment uses the meridians of the large intestines, stomach and lungs with good effect.

Massage

Gentle facial massage helps to drain the sinuses, and in addition relieves headaches by inducing a relaxation effect.

Reflexology

Massage to the reflex areas relating to the nose and sinuses stimulates the healing process.

Homeopathy

- *Arsenicum iodatum*: for symptoms showing a profuse thick yellow discharge
- *Graphites*: where there is an acute sense of smell, and cracks inside the nose
- *Hydrastasis*: used in persistent rhinorrhoea, with burning mucus, a postnasal drip and the presence of small ulcers on the septum
- *Kali bichromium*: used in the presence of lumpy, green catarrh with a feeling of pressure around the bridge of the nose

- *Natrum muriaticum*: for white-looking catarrh with the loss of smell and taste
- *Sanguinaria*: where there is a profuse, offensive, yellow catarrh with frequent sneezing
- *Pulsatilla*: for yellow or green catarrh, which is worse in a warm room

Nasal polyps

Homeopathy

Polypectomy may be avoided by the use of the following homeopathic remedies:

- *Calcarea*: when there is soreness and yellow catarrh
- *Phosphorus*: when polyps bleed easily this remedy is often indicated
- *Psorinum*: for a postnasal drip in a person who is feeling weak and cold
- *Pulsatilla*: indicated in yellow catarrh, which is usually worse in a warm room
- *Sanguinaria*: where there is profuse catarrh and the membranes are dry and hot
- *Thuja*: this is the commonest remedy used where there is chronic catarrh.

Sinusitis

This painful condition is more likely to respond to early intervention. Homeopathy has undergone trials for the treatment of sinusitis.[3]

Acupuncture

The large and small intestine meridians are stimulated to encourage the healing process.

Aromatherapy

Inhalations on a tissue of a few drops of eucalyptus oil, peppermint, lemon, lavender or bergamot are beneficial. A lotion from the same remedies can be used nightly for chronic sinusitis.

Herbal medicine

Steam inhalations of lavender, camomile, pine, eucalyptus and thyme are used. Infusions of ginger, eye bright, peppermint and elderflower may also help. For prevention purposes, garlic can be used on a daily basis.

Reflexology

Areas relating to the sinuses are massaged to induce healing.

Homeopathy

- *Kali bichromium*: for congestion of the nose with stringy catarrh

- *Hepar sulphuris*: the catarrh is yellow, in an irritable and chilly person with sneezing, and for a tender face in a hypersensitive individual
- *Silicea*: this is for predominantly throbbing and tearing facial pain
- *Pulsatilla*: for the presence of yellow catarrh, frontal pain, neuralgia on the right side of the face and where the person is easily reduced to tears
- *Belladonna*: for sudden-onset, fever, red, hot face and where the symptoms are aggravated with the slightest pressure on lying down

---

Case study 25.3

Mabel, a 33-year old non-smoker, presented with a 6-month history of frontal headaches due to sinusitis. These headaches were different from her usual migraine attacks. She felt a pressure in the frontal region. Olbus oil relieved the headaches temporarily only. On examination there was no sinus tenderness in either the maxillary or the frontal areas. She was prescribed Natrum muriaticum and Lycopodium homeopathic remedies. The olbus oil inhalations were discontinued as these interfere with the action of the homeopathic remedies.

Her symptoms had resolved until three months later, when she presented with recurrent frontal sinus headaches, which were quite severe for a week. She was prescribed antibiotics by her own doctor, but this had not resolved the problem, as her sinuses were still tender. Mabel was then prescribed Silicea, a homeopathic remedy, for one week and her symptoms resolved completely. Five months later Silicea and Natrum muriaticum were repeated for a recurrence, with success. Her constitutional remedy, Pulsatilla was then prescribed (*see* Chapter 12). On review 6 months later, she remained well with no recurrence of either the sinusitis or the migraine headaches.

Upper respiratory tract infections

Homeopathy

The use of homeopathy will often reduce the overall rate of antibiotic prescribing (*see* Chapter 12).

- *Aconite napellis*: for sudden onset of symptoms, sneezing, restlessness, which is worse at night, with a burning throat
- *Belladonna*: for the symptoms of fever, flushing, sore throat, cough and thirst
- *Gelsemium*: for flu-like symptoms, shivering and aching with heavy limbs
- *Nux vomica*: usually given to an irritable, critical person who is chilly and has rhinorrhoea during the day only
- *Mercurius*: used where a coated tongue, halitosis, sneezing and a thick yellow–green catarrh are present
- *Hepar sulphuris*: for a sore throat 'as if it had a splinter', otitis media and catarrh which is yellow–green and thick. Usually used in a chilly, irritable and sensitive person

- *Bryonia*: for a patient who has a headache made worse by coughing and where there is a dry mouth, thirst, irritability and the patient wants to be left alone
- *Allium cepa*: for lacrimation, nasal discharge, a burning feeling of the upper lip and where the patient feels better in fresh air
- *Causticum*: used for laryngitis, postnasal drip, dry throat and stress incontinence.

Cold sores
Homeopathy
Homeopathic remedies are used for this acute condition as illustrated. In addition, a constitutional homeopathic remedy can be used to improve the person's immune system to reduce or prevent further attacks (*see* Chapter 12).

- *Capsicum*: for the presence of cracks on the corners of the mouth, an itchy red rash on the chin, with burning blisters on the tongue and halitosis
- *Natrum muriaticum*: usually used for the presence of a crack in the middle of the lower lip and blisters around the lips
- *Rhus toxicodendron*: used where there are ulcers present in the corner of the mouth

Influenza
In influenza, as with all acute conditions, a remedy is given frequently at the onset of treatment, and then less frequently until the infection resolves and is treated symptomatically.

Herbal medicine
Ginger and cinnamon are beneficial herbs as hot teas at the onset of symptoms, elderflower, peppermint and yarrow infusions for the fever stage.

Homeopathy
- *Aconite napellis*: given regularly at the onset of the infection
- *Belladonna*: for a high temperature of sudden onset and in a hot flushed person
- *Bryonia*: for a patient who is hot and irritable, worse especially on movement, and thirsty with headache made worse by coughing.
- *Arsenicum album*: for a pale, chilly, thirsty and anxious person
- *Gelsemium*: used in a person suffering from exhaustion with a bursting headache, which is relieved by urinating
- *Eupatorium*: for limb pains, bursting headache, shivering and where the eyeballs feel sore
- *Pyrogenium*: for myalgia of the thighs, tachycardia and restlessness with only a mild fever
- *Rhus toxicodendron*: for myalgia with extreme restlessness

- *Glonoinum*: for a throbbing, pulsating, bursting type of headache
- *Phytolacca*: used when lymphadenopathy and otalgia are present

---

Case study 25.4

Andrew, a 33 year old, presented with an eight-day history of a flu-like illness. He was at this stage improving, and had developed a dry cough but was still sweating and had lost 3 kg in weight. His dilemma was that 3 days later he was due to run in the London marathon. He had invested months of training and did not want to cancel the run. Andrew was prescribed Arnica 30c twice daily, starting immediately and was to continue taking it until three days after the marathon. He was able to complete the run successfully and did not suffer with any postviral complications as a result.

Glandular fever

Herbal medicine

Infusions of elderflower and yarrow are beneficial for symptomatic relief.

Homeopathy

- *Belladonna*: for patients with a high fever, who are flushed with sudden onset of symptoms
- *Ailanthus*: where there are ulcers in the throat, myalgia, general malaise and headache
- *Cistus*: in a shivery, chilly person with lymph nodes, which are painful on protruding the tongue. It is used for cases where mental exertion makes the symptoms worse
- *Phytolacca*: for patients where swallowing produces an earache, and food and hot drinks make swallowing more painful
- *Calcarea*: for an individual who is sweating and chilly, with a sour taste in the mouth and feeling mentally and physically exhausted
- *Glandular fever nosode*: this can be used in contacts as a means of prevention. In post-glandular fever syndrome, the patient is usually prescribed their constitutional remedy and Glandular fever nosode (*see* Chapter 12).

> *Strive to become a pure being.*
>
> *Geshe Kelsang Gyatso*[4]

References

1   Lambert T, Gresty MA and Bronstein AM. Benign positional vertigo: recognition and treatment. *BMJ* 1995; 311: 489–91.
2   Jacobs J, Springer DA and Crothers D. Homeopathic treatment of acute otitis media in children: a preliminary randomised placebo-controlled trial. *Paediatr Infect Dis J* 2001; 20: 177–83.
3   Weiser M and Clasen BPE. Controlled double-blind study of homeopathic sinusitis medication. *Biol Ther* 1995; 13: 4–11.
4   Gyatso GK. *The New Meditation Handbook.* Ulverston: Tharpa Publications; 2001.

Further reading

•   Harrison H, Fixsen A and Vickers A. A randomised comparison of a homeopathic and standard care for the treatment of glue ear, in children. *Complement Ther Med* 1999; 7: 132–5.

26

Headaches

Just as logic guides the mind desire guides the soul.

Thomas Moore[1]

The main task when dealing with headaches is to separate the causes that can be treated appropriately and safely, by integrating complementary therapies, from causes that need a conventional approach.

As always in medicine there is no substitute for a concise, clear history to enable an accurate diagnosis to be made. It is then possible to identify the minority of headaches presenting that need to be diagnosed and treated urgently. This category includes temporal arteritis, glaucoma, subdural haematoma and bacterial meningitis, where urgent hospital referral for conventional treatment is indicated. Delay in diagnosis and treatment in these conditions can often have serious consequences. Having said this, however, the majority of headaches have a benign cause and are suitable for treatment with many of the complementary therapies.

The following guidelines are included to help differentiate between the more serious causes and the benign headache:

- *age*: headaches arising for the first time in the over 50-years age group are of particular concern. In patients aged over 60 years especially, temporal arteritis, glaucoma and subdural haematoma are a possibility
- *previous history of headaches*
- *length of symptoms*
- *focal neurological symptoms*: where the 'focus' relates to one area of the brain anatomically
- although rare, *remember carbon monoxide poisoning*. Ask if any other member of the family suffers with headache
- *medication*
- *pattern recognition*: the classic example is migraine, which can start at any age.

Causes of headaches

Primary

- Migraine
- Tension headaches
- Cluster headaches
- Others (headaches related to cough for example)

Secondary

- Head or neck trauma
- Head or neck vascular disease (temporal arteritis and aneurysm)
- Head or neck non-vascular (brain tumour)
- Substance/drug use
- Infection
- Homeostatic
- ENT, dental, eye disease
- Neuralgias
- Psychiatric
- Others

Headaches that are suitable for complementary therapies

Primary causes

All **primary** causes of headaches are safe to treat with an integrated approach. Migraine, tension headaches and cluster headaches are suitable conditions.

Homeopathic approach

This outline illustrates the diversity and complexity of tailoring the remedy prescribing to individual patients with headaches.[2]

- *Lachesis*: the patient generally has left-sided headaches
- *Natrum muriaticum*: often used when the pain is described as pulsating
- *Sepia*: for 'hormonal' headaches, for example premenstrual syndrome and the menopause
- *Arnica*: useful for the effects of a head injury
- *Lycopodium*: for right-sided headaches, which are worse between 4 and 8 pm
- *Nux vomica*: for the irritable personality with a headache
- *Pulsatilla*: used in fair-haired women with a gentle temperament

In the treatment of benign headaches, the following are some of the other complementary therapies that can also be used:

- acupuncture (*see* Chapter 7)
- aromatherapy (*see* Chapter 8)
- herbal medicine (*see* Chapter 11)
- reflexology (*see* Chapter 18)
- Reiki (*see* Chapter 19)
- remedial massage (*see* Chapter 14)
- yoga (*see* Chapter 21).

Secondary causes

In **secondary** causes of headaches, there are some conditions that are appropriate for using an integrated approach.

In head and neck trauma the following can be helpful.

Homeopathy
- *Arnica*: often used to relieve bruising pain
- *Rhus toxicodendron*: this is especially useful for pain that improves on movement

Acupuncture
This treatment can help alleviate pain particularly if it becomes a chronic problem.

Osteopathy and remedial massage
This may be considered for pain relief to help relax the muscles.

Reiki
This can often help with 'post-trauma' tension, and produces a relaxation effect.

Physiotherapy/massage
This can often be of help and integrates well with complementary therapies.

Acute and chronic sinusitis are amenable to homeopathic treatment (*see* Chapter 25). Neuralgias in particular may respond to acupuncture and homeopathy (*see* Chapter 23). For psychiatric and emotional causes, the root problem needs to be identified and the headache treated holistically. If stress, depression or bereavement is the underlying problem these must be addressed accordingly (*see* Chapters 3, 4 and 6).

> *Words of affirmation will always create an atmosphere in your home that's conducive to calm and repose.*
>
> *Titus 3:8*

References

1 Moore T. *Care of the Soul. A Guide for Cultivating Depth and Sacredness in Everyday Life*. New York: HarperCollins; 1992.
2 Brigo B and Serpelloni G. Homeopathic treatment of migraines: a randomised double-blind controlled study of sixty cases (homeopathic remedy versus placebo). *Berlin J Res Homeopath* 1991; 1: 98–106.

Further reading

- Davenport RJ. Sudden headache in the emergency department. *Pract Neurol* 2005; 5; 132–43.
- Packard RC. What does the headache patient want? *Headache* 1979; 19: 370–4.

Contacts

- *International Headache Society*: www.i-h-s.org

27

Obstetrics and gynaecology

Love alone is capable of uniting living beings in such a way as to complete and fulfil them, for it alone takes them and joins them by what is deepest in themselves ... and if that is what it can achieve daily on a small scale, why should it not repeat this one day on worldwide dimensions?

Pierre Teilhard De Chardin[1]

The aim always in antenatal care is to avoid using medication in treating the mother that may harm the foetus. Most complementary therapies are ideal as they are safe and free from side-effects. Homeopathy, acupuncture and the touch therapies, in particular, are effective in treating premenstrual and menopausal women, alleviating many distressing symptoms. Details of each therapy are in the relevant chapters.

Antenatal care

The following therapies are beneficial in treating women with antenatal problems:

- acupuncture
- herbal medicine
- massage
- reflexology
- Reiki
- homeopathy
- meditation
- yoga.

These therapies help in relaxation, which in turn reduces labour pains, improves contractions and contributes to a healthy outcome in intrapartum care. Homeopathy and acupuncture are described, to show the role of these therapies in integration.

Homeopathy

Caulophyllum is prescribed weekly, from 32 weeks' gestation until delivery. This aids smooth contractions at the time of labour. For perinatal care, Arnica and Hypericum are given for pain relief. These remedies are also given at the onset of labour and continued for a few days afterwards, especially following an episiotomy or Caesarean section. During the antenatal period, most acute conditions can be treated with homeopathic remedies, making it safe for the mother and the baby, avoiding any side-effects. Haemorrhoids, for example, can be treated with Pulsatilla, Nux vomica, Arsenicum and Carbo vegetabilis. Anal fissures can be treated effectively with Apis mellifica and/or Silica and topical Calendula cream.

Acupuncture

In pregnancy, acupuncture has been used for pain relief during labour, backache and pain relief in general. A prospective, quasi-randomised controlled trial concluded that the study suggested that acupuncture alleviates insomnia during pregnancy.[2]

A study was conducted on the relief of low back pain in pregnancy, using acupuncture in 61 women.[3] The women were allocated randomly into two groups, those treated by acupuncture and a control group. Twenty-seven patients formed the study group, and 34 the control group. The severity of pain was measured using a numerical rating scale from 0 to 10. The use of conventional analgesic drugs was also assessed. Women were followed up for eight weeks at two-weekly intervals. The average pain scores decreased by 50% in 21 (78%) patients in the acupuncture group, and in 5 (15%) patients in the control group, thus reducing the need for drugs, which is an advantage in pregnancy.[3]

Morning sickness

This symptom can be very distressing and debilitating in early pregnancy.

Herbal medicine

Regular infusions of tea made with fresh ginger, peppermint or camomile at regular intervals help relieve nausea.

Homeopathy

- *Ipecacuanha*: can be taken regularly for constant nausea and vomiting
- *Argentum nitricum*: used for anxiety, panic and a craving for sweet food
- *Sepia*: used for sadness and indifference
- *Pulsatilla*: used for tearfulness, feeling better for fresh air and aggravated by fatty foods
- *Nux vomica*: for nausea that is worse in the morning, with irritability

Gynaecology

Infertility

Many couples, after investigations for fertility, are found to be healthy and well with no physical reason for their problems. Stress is a recognised cause of infertility; complementary therapies help relaxation and indirectly aid conception. General preconceptual advice on lifestyle, exercise, nutrition and folic acid supplements are important. Any symptoms of premenstrual syndrome can also be treated in the same way, avoiding drugs in women during the preconceptual and conceptual parts of the menstrual cycle.

Dysmenorrhoea

Spasmodic dysmenorrhoea responds well to the homeopathic remedy Magnesia phosphorica and the herb Agnus castus. If premenstrual syndrome is also present and contributing to the dysmenorrhoea, then this can be treated in order to alleviate the pain.

For secondary causes, such as endometriosis, laparoscopic investigation will confirm the diagnosis and there is often also associated infertility. The pain can be managed with homeopathic remedies (*see* Chapter 12). Therapies for stress relief can also be used: acupuncture (*see* Chapter 7), Reiki (*see* Chapter 19) and meditation (*see* Chapter 15).

Menorrhagia

Examination and investigation are essential for an accurate diagnosis to determine the cause of menorrhagia. Fibroids, pelvic inflammatory disease, endometriosis, endometrial polyps and dysfunctional uterine bleeding can be the underlying cause.

Homeopathy (see Chapter 12)

The remedies Sepia, Pulsatilla, Agnus castus, Sulphur and Lillium tigrinum can relieve menorrhagia, and a constitutional remedy may also be added.

Premenstrual syndrome

Premenstrual syndrome (PMS) affects women of childbearing years and is a very common condition. By definition, it is the cyclical recurrence of symptoms for three months or more. The symptoms can begin up to two weeks before the start of menstruation and usually settle within the first few days of menstruation. Fluid retention with weight gain, mastalgia, bloating, irritability, headaches, sleep disturbance and changes in libido are common symptoms. Often, chronic conditions such as asthma, depression, migraine and irritable bowel syndrome can be exacerbated with PMS. Sustained stress often triggers the condition. Hormonal changes with the combined oral contraceptive pill can also be a cause due to a relative deficiency in vitamin B_6 (pyridoxine). The cyclical symptoms can be mild, moderate or severe, causing considerable disruption in a woman's life during the premenstrual phase. Mood swings can be associated with relatively low blood sugar levels, and the management of PMS must always involve dietary adjustment.

Dietary advice

A 3-hourly carbohydrate diet will ensure blood sugar levels are maintained, reducing headaches and mood swings quite significantly. Dietary changes alone can often improve up to 50% of the symptoms of premenstrual syndrome (*see* Chapter 22).

Herbal medicine (see Chapter 11)

Evening primrose oil can be bought over the counter and works well in this condition, taken for at least three months.

Stress management

Stress relief is essential to help the mind and body to rest and relax to produce peace of mind (*see* Chapter 3) and relieve the symptoms.

Reiki

See Chapter 19.

Reflexology

See Chapter 18.

Aromatherapy

See Chapter 8.

Meditation

See Chapter 15.

Exercise

See Chapter 22.

Massage

See Chapter 14.

Acupuncture

See Chapter 7.

These are all balancing and relaxing tools to help the body to achieve optimum benefits and emotional and physical relief, stimulate the immune system and increase a feeling of 'wellbeing'.

Homeopathy

- *Lachesis*: used in chilly, pale, talkative women whose symptoms settle at onset of menses
- *Natrum muriaticum*: for women who have mood swings, prefer savoury food and are tearful
- *Pulsatilla*: for a gentle personality who is easily weepy and with a late menarche
- *Sepia*: for exhausted, pale women who are chilly and not thirsty

Cystitis

Cystitis is a very common bladder problem most often associated with women. It arises mainly because of the anatomical location of the urethral opening in the vulva area and the perineum, which are in close proximity to the anus. Cystitis is the term for burning, irritation and frequency symptoms that can cause much pain and distress. This condition often has an associated dull pain in the lower abdomen. Antibiotics may be used if appropriate. The use of complementary therapies may well avoid antibiotic treatment. A midstream specimen of urine can be cultured to check the effectiveness of whichever treatment is used.

Urethral syndrome

This is chronic irritation of the urethra and bladder as a result of:

- contraception
- hormone imbalance
- an allergic reaction
- sexual intercourse.

Medical management of cystitis usually results in antibiotic treatment, however using an integrated approach can minimise this.

Homeopathy

- *Staphysagria*: for frequency with stinging, cutting pains
- *Cantharis*: this is useful in dysuria and urgency
- *Belladonna*: for dysuria and when there are blood clots present
- *Causticum*: used when there is a vaginal discharge and frequency of micturition
- *Sarsaparilla*: used in cases where there is a milky-looking urine with urgency

Self-help

- Increase fluids to flush out the infection and if possible 500 ml hourly, initially.
- Reduce the acidity of fluids ingested by adding barley water.
- Use Cranberry juice for prevention, advise one glass twice a day.
- If an antibiotic is used, include natural live yogurt (containing lactobacillus) to replace the bowel flora in the diet on a daily basis.
- Empty the bladder regularly.
- Wear only natural fibre underwear such as cotton.
- Use non-perfumed soap, vaginal deodorants and bath oils.
- Avoid using tampons.
- Change underwear regularly.
- Do not wash underwear in biological powder or bleach.
- Sexual intercourse: drink about 500 ml of water before and after intercourse.
- Urinate before and directly after sexual intercourse (both partners should wash before).

Menopause

Many women in the west equate the menopause with having a medical condition that requires treatment. It is deemed as a negative part of life, not the gift it really is. The age group affected usually ranges from the early 40s up to the mid 50s. It is often associated with a lack of femininity, lost youth and redundant sex life, and usually coincides with the 'empty nest syndrome'.

In other parts of the world it is not really an issue, it is perceived as a natural event and hormone replacement therapy (HRT) is rarely prescribed. Women in India, for example, feel that there are many advantages as they receive much greater respect, so it is something to look forward to. African women receive a much higher status in the community as they reach the menopause, taking a more active role in decision making outside the home. American women on the other hand see the menopause as the beginning of the ageing process, in terms of looks, and something to be dreaded.

The menopause is a gradual process of maturing and letting go of the past and looking forward to the future, a redefining of roles and life stages. A woman's individual perspective returns, having received the freedom from children, parents and fear of pregnancy and and being able to spend more time with her partner. It is time to take stock and do all those things that the family and time did not allow. Women are now much more empowered to find ways of dealing with the more troublesome symptoms. A number of treatments exist to manage this phase of the female lifecycle and can be tailored to individual needs.

Symptoms of the menopause

For some women there is only slight discomfort, while for others the effect is quite debilitating during this phase. The symptoms can affect women emotionally, physically and psychologically.

Some of the distressing symptoms experienced during the menopause are:

- anxiety
- depression
- insomnia
- lack of concentration
- mood swings
- forgetfulness
- palpitations
- loss of bladder control
- hair loss
- headaches
- back pain
- night sweats
- hot flushes
- dry skin
- loss of libido
- vulval pruritus
- dyspareunia
- dryness of the hair and eyes

- bloated abdomen
- facial hair
- mastalgia
- constipation.

Management of the menopause

Management depends on the presenting symptoms.

Hormone replacement therapy

If taken for more than 5 years, HRT increases the risk of breast cancer.[4] The prevention and treatment of osteoporosis and the role of HRT is well researched.[5]

Homeopathy

Remedies are tailored to the individual. Some of the more common remedies used are:

- *Sulphur*: this helps relieve hot flushes
- *Graphites*: for weight gain with red face, and cracks in the skin
- *Lachesis*: for fluid retention, and talkative woman with hot flushes
- *Sepia*: this patient often has dryness of the vagina with uterine prolapse
- *Agnus castus*: regularly used for PMS with pain and tearfulness
- *Bryonia*: effective for mastalgia
- *Vervain*: helpful for fluctuating emotions and anxiety
- *Cimcifuja*: used for muscle aches and pains with intercostal myalgia
- *Avena sativa*: useful for sleep disturbance and to calm the whole system

Herbal medicine (see Chapter 11)

The following herbs are beneficial for symptom relief:

- *Black cohosh and Agnus castus*: both of these herbs work well together and are thought to have oestrogenic properties (*see* Chapter 11)
- *Alfalfa*: mineral replacement, calcium and oestrogenic properties
- *Sage*: available in tea and tablet form, useful for hot flushes
- *St John's wort*: for depression, insomnia and poor memory (*see* Chapter 11)
- *Wild yam*: thought to help increase hormone levels
- *Vervain*: indicated in anxiety and restlessness.

Relaxation

Yoga (*see* Chapter 21), massage (*see* Chapter 14), meditation (*see* Chapter 15) and hobbies are all helpful. These help the mind and body keep the balance as the hormone levels are decreasing, and to improve sleep patterns and induce relaxation.

Exercise

Regular walking and swimming for example are easy to do and help tone the muscles and increase the 'feel good factor' (*see* Chapter 22).

Aromatherapy (see Chapter 8)

Some of the common remedies that can be obtained in many local shops include:

- *Basil*: for tiredness
- *Lavender and Neroli*: used in insomnia
- *Rose, Sage and Clary*: for depression
- *Avocado and Wheatgerm*: for dry skin
- *Cypress and Geranium*: for menorrhagia.

Nutritional balance

Regular meals help to reduce mood swings, with added fresh fruits and vegetables to increase fibre. Hot spicy foods should be avoided, as these will aggravate vasomotor problems such as night sweats and flushing. Increase fluid intake (water 2 litres daily), and a reduction in tea, coffee and alcohol will also help (*see* Chapter 22).

Supplements (see Chapter 22)

- Calcium, Zinc, Vitamin B, Magnesium, Omega 3 and Evening primrose oil
- For vaginal dryness, oestrogen cream, Replens and for external use KY jelly and baby oil.

Case study 27.1

June, a 50 year old, complained of postmenopausal bleeding, 2 years after her last menstrual period. She was referred for gynaecological investigation. A hysteroscopy, dilatation and curettage were performed, and no pathology was found. The cause was diagnosed as atrophic vaginitis. Homeopathic Pulsatilla was prescribed, which improved her symptoms considerably. As she still had some residual vaginitis, a small amount of oestrogen cream twice weekly was applied sparingly. She improved over the following months, repeating the Pulsatilla every few months to keep her symptoms under control. This demonstrates good integration and appropriate joint care with her gynaecologist and family doctor/homeopathic physician.

Our true home is in the present moment.
To live in the present moment is a miracle.
The miracle is not to walk on water.
The miracle is to walk on the green Earth in the present moment.
Daniel J O'Leary[6]

References

1 De Chardin PT. *Hymn of the Universe*. New York: Harper and Row; 1965.
2 da Silva JBG, Nakamura MU, Cordeiro JA *et al*. Acupuncture for insomnia in pregnancy – a prospective, quasi-randomised controlled study. *Acupunct Med* 2005; 23: 47–51.
3 da Silva JBG, Nakamura MU, Cordeiro JA *et al*. Acupuncture for low back-pain in pregnancy – a prospective, quasi-randomised, controlled study. *Acupunct Med* 2004; 22: 60–7.
4 Beral V, Banks E and Reeves G. Evidence from randomised trials on the long-term effects of hormone replacement therapy. *Lancet* 2002; 360: 942–4.
5 Wimalawansa SJ. A four-year randomised controlled trial of hormone replacement and biphosphonate, alone or in combination, in women with postmenopausal osteoporosis. *Am J Med* 1998: 104: 219–26.
6 O'Leary DJ. *Travelling Light. Your Journey to Wholeness*. Dublin: The Columba Press; 2001.

Further reading

• Darnell P, Pinder M and Treacy K (eds). *Searching for Evidence: complementary therapies research*. London. The Prince of Wales Foundation for Integrated Health, 2006.
• Demetriou A. Counselling after miscarriage. *Audit Gen Pract* 1995; 3: 18–19.

Contacts

• *Women's Nutritional Advisory Service*: PO Box 268, Lowes, East Sussex BN7 1QN; tel: 01273 487 366
• *National Osteoporosis Society*: www.nos.org.uk; Manor Farm, Skinners Hill, Camerton, Bath BA2 0PJ; tel: 01761 471 771

28

Paediatric medicine

If there is anything we wish to change in the child, we should first examine and see whether it is not something that could better be changed in ourselves.

CG Jung[1]

In children particularly, it is essential that an accurate diagnosis is made to ensure correct and appropriate treatment on the grounds of safety. Whether it is a simple upper respiratory infection, teething or otitis media, it is always imperative that more serious pathology is considered. Children have the capacity to get better very quickly, but equally can become ill very quickly. Parents' instincts and observation must always be taken into account. This cannot be emphasised enough, especially in conditions as serious as meningococcal disease. Doctors and parents on a constant 'alert' can be life saving. At the same time it is important to keep a sensible balance; the basic principle initially is 'common things commonest.'

Complementary therapies

In the diseases that follow, some of the therapies will be discussed, demonstrating how they can be used with good effect and are safe and acceptable in children of all ages.

With homeopathic treatment of infections such as scarlet fever (*see* Chapter 12), the remedies are palatable and avoid causing further gastric irritation from either the infection or conventional medicines. Antibiotics, for example, often add to or induce vomiting and/or diarrhoea in a child who is already ill. This is distressing and can contribute to dehydration. In upper respiratory tract infections, antibiotics are often used inappropriately, even though 90% of such infections are viral. By choosing to use homeopathy, the remedy is given on the basis of the presenting symptoms. If a flushed, feverish child has a viral or bacterial infection, the prescribed remedy is based on the signs and symptoms and can avoid the use of antibiotics. Homeopathic remedies can be given as granules for very young children or tablets sublingually for older children. Using a remedy over the course of a few hours or days will resolve the infection without the need for conventional drugs. In primary care, the use of homeopathy is ideal for common conditions and parents can be taught how to use the remedies for future similar infections and, of course, to seek medical advice when in doubt. Parents are often pleased to do this for the common ailments and many have homeopathic remedy kits at home.

Unnecessary antibiotic prescribing contributes to long-term antibiotic resistance.

Infantile colic

This symptom is very common and distressing for mother and child. Having 'winded' the baby the pain continues. This often occurs when both are tired in the early evening.

Homeopathy

Colocynth is available in granular form and is the commonest remedy prescribed for this condition.

Osteopathy

Cranio-osteopathy is a safe hands-on touch technique effective for colic (*see* Chapter 16).

Teething

This is a very distressing symptom for infants. Homeopathic treatment is an alternative to conventional analgesics and local applications for pain relief.

Homeopathy

- *Calcareum carbonicum*: this remedy is indicated in babies with a birth weight of over 4.5 kg who are often overweight and are 'head sweaters'
- *Chamomilla*: used in an irritable child who wants to be carried, one cheek is red and hot, the other pale when teething.
- *Silica*: used in a thin child, with a 'big' head in proportion to body size, with sweating of the head and feet
- *Colocynth*: for red sore gums, in a fretful and colicky child
- *Belladonna*: a common remedy for red and throbbing sore gums

Threadworms (pinworms)

Homeopathic treatment for threadworms can be used in children of any age, even in infants. A hygiene review of the whole family is essential to prevent further infestation.

Homeopathy

- *Cina*: this is the usual and effective remedy, although others may need to be prescribed when necessary

Herbal medicine

Regular doses of garlic and increased carrot intake have proven effective for worms.

Childhood infections

Complementary remedies are more palatable in children than conventional drugs.

Otitis media

Homeopathy (see Chapter 12)

- *Aconite napellis*: used in a restless, anxious, child at the onset of the illness
- *Belladonna*: used in a child, with a flushed, hot face, fever, and usually sensitive to touch; this remedy usually follows Aconite napellis
- *Pulsatilla*: for, a clingy, weepy child, with earache

Upper respiratory tract infections

Examples are laryngitis, tonsillitis, pharyngitis and coryza.

Homeopathy

- *Aconite napellis*: for sudden onset of symptoms
- *Dulcamara*: used when infection starts after exposure to damp or cold, or after exertion
- *Gelsemium*: used in children who have an unpleasant-tasting mouth, earache, neck ache, are weak and exhausted and are unwilling to take fluids
- *Apis*: for a dry, red, painful, throat

Gastroenteritis

In infants, it is particularly important to ensure enough fluid is tolerated, otherwise admission to hospital for rehydration is essential.

Homeopathy

- *Arsenicum*: indicated in a cold, weak, restless child
- *Colocynth*: for children presenting with colicky abdominal pain with the legs drawn and where slight pressure can relieve the pain
- *Nux vomica*: used for copious diarrhoea and vomiting
- *Phosphoric acid*: useful in diarrhoea with undigested food, where the child seems better for passing stool

Table 28.1 Homeopathic treatment of common childhood infectious diseases

Childhood infection	Homeopathic remedies (see Chapter 12)
Chickenpox	Rhus toxicodendron, Sulphur, Mercurius, Pulsatilla, Antimonium tartaricum
Mumps	Belladonna, Pilocarpine muriaticum, Phytolacca, Mercurius
Measles	Morbilium, Euphrasia, Belladonna, Aconite napellis, Pulsatilla, Bryonia, Sulphur
Glandular fever	Belladonna, Cistus, Phytolacca, Baryta carbonica, Calcarea, Mercurius
Warts	Thuja, Causticum, Nitric acid, Calcarea, Antimonium crudum, Dulcamara, Kali muriaticum, Natrum carbonicum

Asthma

Integrating complementary treatment in asthma must be approached initially by continuing any conventional medicine already prescribed. The homeopathic, herbal, acupuncture or other therapy can then be introduced. Eventually, conventional drugs can be reduced gradually as the asthma is controlled. This then becomes a safe way to manage the disease. In this instance, integrated care means that in a chronic disease such as asthma, complementary remedies are used to alleviate symptoms, but where this is not possible then the aim is to use less of the conventional drugs. The patient's response to complementary therapies can be assessed and conventional medication adjusted accordingly. Often complementary therapies on their own will suffice, and sometimes both complementary and conventional medicines are needed. Monitoring the asthma is, therefore, important.

Homeopathy

Remedies are used in relieving the symptoms in an acute or chronic situation. In addition, there is also a desensitising role to try and control the long-term fluctuations of asthma.[2–4] There are remedies made from horse, cat and dog hair, which are used over a period of weeks to desensitise an individual with a history of one of these allergies. Homeopathic remedies, which can be used in acute exacerbation of asthma include Sambucus, Arsenicum, Carbo vegetabilis, Ipecacuanha, Nux vomica, Phosphorus, Kali carbonicum, Natrum sulphuricum, Chamomilla, Pulsatilla and Aconite napellis.

House dust mite control

Emphasis is also placed on the control of house dust mite within the home. Parents are taught to vacuum and wet dust the child's bedroom daily for 6 weeks. Also, any covers and bedding are shaken outside the house as much as possible to remove surface dust. The house dust mite has a 6-week cycle; after this period of intensive cleaning, maintenance two to three times a week is also advised. Pillows or quilts with feathers are also removed from the bedroom; this can help control the asthma by reducing the allergens.

Eczema (see adult eczema; Chapter 24)

Behavioural problems

In bedwetting, autism, attention deficit syndrome, breath-holding attacks, clumsiness, dyslexia and febrile convulsions, homeopathic treatment is helpful and will need an assessment by a qualified homeopath. Remedies can be used in conjunction with conventional and psychological techniques.

Integrated health care in paediatric pain management

In 2005 a survey of major universities in the US was conducted examining the use of complementary therapies for paediatric pain management. Forty-three paediatric anaesthetic fellowship programmes (100%) responded to the survey. Thirty-eight institutions (86%) offered one or more therapies for their patients.[5]

Those therapies included:

- biofeedback (65%)
- visualisation (49%)
- relaxation therapy (33%)
- massage (35%)
- hypnosis (44%)
- acupuncture (33%)
- art therapy (21%)
- meditation (21%).

This illustrates the high prevalence of the integration of complementary medicine into paediatric pain management programmes in the USA.

Children, healthy eating and lifestyle

Healthy lifestyles and dietary habits have a major bearing on children's 'wellbeing'. Living and eating habits have changed quite significantly without enough importance being placed on the effects on the long-term health of children.[6,7] Society has become very fast-food orientated. The food industry is certainly thriving, as children in particular are bombarded with foods that have higher levels of additives, preservatives, colourings, salt, sugar and fats. It is fairly common to see children with a packet of crisps or a bottle of fizzy drink; it is rare to see children with fruit in their hand. The Food Standards Agency (FSA) conducted a national diet and nutrition survey of 5–18 year olds, which showed that young people are eating:[8]

- too much saturated fat: 14.3% of food energy (the recommended level is 11%)
- too much sugar: added sugar provides 16.5% of food energy (the recommended level is 11%)
- too little fruit: average consumption of fruit and vegetables was 2–3 portions, one in five children eat no fruit at all
- too few vitamins and minerals: 42% of teenage girls are not getting enough iron, 13% of all teenagers are low in vitamin D.

Children are growing up with very little knowledge or skills relating to the basics of healthy eating. No longer are they expected to help prepare a meal for the family. Modern lifestyle has become much more frenetic and more pressured, quality time with children is limited, and the 'takeaway' is an easier option. This is fine as a treat, but not on a regular basis. The FSA concluded that 'healthy choices should be easy choices'.[8] Parents have a responsibility to choose healthy food, which should be readily available and affordable. Food awareness should start in the home, be taught in schools as an essential part of the curriculum, and be included in parenting classes. The dietary advice and needs of the population are the responsibility of the food industry, government, the media and the health service. The food that our children consume is a collective responsibility if we are to help prevent disease and ensure healthy balanced adults.

Management of nutrition and lifestyle in children must include the whole family.

A healthy balanced diet should include three meals a day with at least five portions of fruit and vegetables, for example:

- baked/boiled potatoes instead of fried
- increased fluid intake/water
- healthy snacks
- increased fibre
- more fish and chicken
- reduced sugar intake.

This should include a family meal at least once a day (for health and communication purposes).

Exercise

This should be family orientated to show an example to children, such as regular swimming, walking, football, and other outdoor activities (*see* Chapter 22). Exercise must be taken more seriously as an integral part of prevention and health promotion.

Relaxation

Relaxation should be a normal part of gaining life skills. Some schools now embrace meditation and yoga as a tool for helping to calm the mind and help concentration. Hobbies and physical activities should be encouraged, which will help children to relax, thus improving perspective. Relaxation is a skill that requires practice like any other as part of everyday life. Children need to embrace this early to learn to take responsibility for their own health promotion as adults.

Childhood obesity

With the increase in childhood and adolescent obesity in the UK the fact is that adult males have one of the highest obesity rates in Europe. We do not have a choice but to take these statistics of this major health threat seriously. Up to 75% of obese children become obese adults, carrying their risk factors and co-morbidities with them.[6] The health risks of childhood obesity are also associated with increased blood pressure, dyslipidaemia and left ventricular hypertrophy. There is an increasing prevalence of type 2 diabetes in children, and one-quarter of these fulfil the criteria for the metabolic syndrome.[6] Attempts are being made to stem the tide of childhood obesity by treating each child individually. A current successful initiative in childhood obesity is MEND, (M)ind (E)xercise, (N)utrition and (D)iet and is both evidence based and outcome driven. MEND is based at the Great Ormond Street Hospital in London and run by a multidisciplinary team. It is community and family based, for overweight and obese children aged between 7 and 12 years and their families.[7]

Homeopathy and immunisation in children

The national immunisation programme is constantly being updated. This important prevention programme is in place to protect all children, and a high uptake is necessary for an effective public health policy. All vaccinations rely on achieving adequate antibody levels to protect an individual. To date, the current knowledge is that the immunisation programme is safe for the majority of children. The use of 'alternatives' such as homeopathy has never been shown to raise antibody levels, and therefore cannot be recommended to protect children against infectious diseases. There are no *proven* homeopathic substitutes for immunisation. The Faculty of Homeopathy, in fact, follows and recommends the Department of Health Guidelines on immunisation in the normal way unless there are medical contraindications. Homeopathy can be an appropriate way to treat the ill-effects of immunisation. In children who have contraindication to immunisation and succumb to infectious diseases, then homeopathy can be used as a treatment.

Maturing means regaining the seriousness we had as children at play.

Friedrich Nietzsche[9]

References

1 Jung CG. *Collected Works. Volume 8*. London: Routledge Kegan Paul; 1970.
2 Poitevin B. Review of experimental studies in allergy: clinical studies. *Br Homeopath J* 1998; 87: 89–99.
3 Gnaiger J. Allergic asthma. *Br Homeopath J* 1990; 79: 135–7.
4 Eizayaga FX, Eizayaga J and Eizayaga FX. Homoeopathic treatment of bronchial asthma, retrospective study of 62 cases. *Br Homoeopath J* 1996; 85: 28–33.
5 Lin Y, Lee A, Kemper K *et al*. Use of complementary and alternative medicine in paediatric pain management service: a survey. *Pain Med* 2005; 6: 452–8.
6 Haslam D. What's new – Tackling Childhood Obesity Symposium – paediatric medicine. *Practitioner* 2006: 250: 26–35.
7 Sacher PM, Chadwick P, Wells JCK *et al*. Assessing the acceptability and feasibility of the MEND Programme in a small group of obese 7–11-year-old children. *J Hum Nutr Dietet* 2005; 18: 3–5.
8 Food Standards Agency. www.food.gov.uk (accessed 15 October 2006).
9 Nietzsche FW. *The Complete Works of Friedrich Nietzsche*. Stanford, CA: Stanford University Press; 1995.

Further reading

- Davies S and Stewart A. *Nutritional Medicine. The drug free guide to better family health*. London: Pan Books; 1987.
- Eckersley J. *Coping with Childhood Allergies*. London: Sheldon Press; 2005.
- Erikson E. *Childhood and Society*. New York: WW Norton; 1964, p. 259.
- Keston D. *Feeding the Body, Nourishing the Soul*. London: Conari Press; 1997.

Contacts

- *Food Matter*: www.foodmatter.com; 5 Lawn Road, London NW3 2XS
- *The National Institute of Medical Herbalists*: www.nimh.org.uk; www.mynutrition.co.uk; Elm House, 54 Mary Arches Street, Exeter, Devon EX4 3BA; tel: 01392 426022
- *Childhood Obesity Guidelines*: www.nationalobesityforum.org.uk; www.healthforallchildren. co.uk; www.mendprogramme.com

29

Palliative care

Once you have found yourself,
you have found your home,
you have found the love,
you have found your,
inexhaustible ecstasy
you have found the whole
of existence is ready for you,
to dance, to rejoice, and to sing –
to live intensively and to die
blissfully. These things happen
of their own accord.

Osho[1]

Palliative care is the active holistic care of patients with advanced, progressive illness. Management of pain and other symptoms, and the provision of psychological, social and spiritual support are paramount. The goal of palliative care is the achievement of the best quality of life for patients and their families. Many aspects of palliative care are also applicable earlier in the course of the illness in conjunction with other treatments.[2]

The principles and aims of palliative care are to:

- affirm life, and regard dying as a natural process
- provide relief from pain and other symptoms
- integrate the psychological and spiritual aspects of care
- offer a support system to help patients live as actively as possible until death
- offer a support system to help the family cope during the patient's illness and their own bereavement.

Integration, complementary therapies and palliative care

The main aspects of palliative care are comprehensively documented in *National Guidelines for the Use of Complementary Therapies in Supportive and Palliative Care*.[2] The report includes guidance on setting up a service in cancer care and sharing the experience in centres of excellence in the UK. Many oncology hospitals and hospices already have an established and flourishing service. Some districts also use community complementary therapy services that are available to cancer and palliative care patients. The most commonly used therapies in palliative care are discussed in outline. Further information is available on each therapy in the relevant chapters.

Acupuncture

This is used increasingly in cancer for pain and symptom control:[2]

- *acute postoperative pain*
- *chronic pain*: the more advanced the cancer the shorter the response to the treatment usually. A study showed pain relief for cancer and a range of other symptoms in which 86% of patients considered the acupuncture service to be very important[3,4]
- *nausea and vomiting*: a number of studies showed positive results when acupuncture was compared with a control group[5]
- *shortness of breath*: a pilot study of 20 patients with breathlessness related to cancer, who were treated with acupuncture, found that 70% improved[6]
- *xerostomia*: acupuncture helped 50% of patients (who were refractory to pilocarpine) with this symptom in one study. It has been shown that acupuncture increases salivary flow[7]
- *hot flushes*: both in the climacteric and in the use of tamoxifen in breast cancer, acupuncture has been shown to reduce hot flushes[8]
- *anxiety and depression*: in anxiety particularly, acupuncture has been shown to be effective with the patient in control of the needles
- *intractable hiccups*: these can be painful and distressing; a study has shown acupuncture to be very successful in symptom relief.[9]

Medical awareness of acupuncture in cancer care

- Avoid spinal areas of instability due to cancer invasion. This can potentially increase the risk of cord compression.
- Do not insert needles over the tumour or ascites.
- Do not use in clotting disorders.
- Avoid indwelling acupuncture needles in immunocompromised patients and those with heart valve disease, to avoid risk of bacteraemia.
- Avoid needles in intracranial deficits following neurosurgery.
- Lymphoedema in limbs should not have needles inserted.
- Avoid needles placed over a prosthesis.

Serious adverse effects of acupuncture

- Trauma to tissues and organs
- Missed or delayed diagnosis by masking symptoms
- Pneumothorax
- Infection: bacterial, viral, hepatitis B, C and HIV. Single-use disposable needles have reduced the spread of hepatitis

Homeopathy

The following symptoms can be alleviated by the use of homeopathic remedies:

- hot flushes
- anxiety and stress
- depression

- fatigue
- skin reactions related to radiotherapy
- postoperative ileus.

Details of the approach in homeopathy and the choice of remedies in alleviating a clinical symptom-complex (cluster of symptoms) are discussed in Chapter 12.

Case study 29.1

Irini, a 56 year old, was diagnosed with invasive ductal carcinoma of the right breast following routine mammography screening. Needle biopsy confirmed advanced carcinoma. A right simple mastectomy was performed the following month, tamoxifen was commenced and in addition Iscador (Mistletoe) injections were given into the right chest area, subcutaneously.[10] Both of these treatments were continued for 10 years. Natrum muriaticum homeopathic remedy was given monthly for 4 months to alleviate her anxiety and depression soon after the diagnosis was made. Now aged 71, and 15 years since the breast cancer was diagnosed, she is in very good health. The mastectomy scar was 'clear'. There was no evidence of recurrence and no lymphadenopathy noted in the axillae, also there was no hepatomegaly. The left breast was normal on palpation. This lady continues to lead a full and normal life, enjoying frequent travels abroad.

Hypnotherapy

Hypnotherapy can be used in conjunction with conventional psychotherapy. One study showed that 70% of patients had greater improvement than those receiving cognitive–behavioural therapy alone.[11] It was also found that the use of hypnotherapy prior to surgery, chemotherapy, radiotherapy and bone marrow transplants can reduce anxiety and the side-effects of treatment.[12]

Hypnotherapy can help in the following conditions:

- nausea and vomiting related to chemotherapy
- prior to surgery
- anxiety and depression in relation to cancer
- pain relief
- immune system response: this is due to improved psychological status. A 10-year randomised trial with 86 women with cancer who received weekly group therapy, showed increased survival rates from recurrence to subsequent death[13]
- to improve quality of life
- to induce a feeling of relaxation and wellbeing.

Contraindications to hypnotherapy

- Underlying psychiatric conditions, which may be exacerbated causing an unpredictable response
- Special care needs to be taken in patients with clinical depression

Touch therapies

- Aromatherapy (*see* Chapter 8)
- Massage (*see* Chapter 14)
- Reflexology (*see* Chapter 18)
- Reiki energy healing (*see* Chapter 19)

These touch therapies are very beneficial in palliative care for:[14,15]

- anxiety
- depression
- inducing relaxation
- emotional and spiritual support
- helping to improve sleep patterns
- reduction of stress, by providing support
- pain reduction and control
- controlling nausea and other side-effects of chemotherapy
- improving the quality of the final stages of life
- supporting the patient generally in palliative care and through the dying process.

Awareness and precautions for hands-on therapies

- Avoid a limb with deep vein thrombosis.
- Avoid areas of bone metastases and use only very gentle strokes.
- Avoid stoma sites, catheters and dressings.
- Use only light pressure over the cancer site.
- In patients who are anticoagulated or have thrombocytopaenia, only light touch should be applied.
- In lymphoedema of limbs, a therapist should work in conjunction with a physiotherapist.
- For ascites, gentle strokes only should be applied.
- Touch therapies are contraindicated in patients with a fever.

> *Eternity is the everlasting now.*
>
> *Johannes Tauler (1291–1361)*

References

1 Osho. *Autobiography of a Spiritually Incorrect Mystic*. New York: St Martin's Press; 2000.
2 Tavares M. *National Guidelines for the Use of Complementary Therapies in Supportive and Palliative Care*. London: The Prince of Wales Foundation for Integrated Health and the National Council for Hospice and Specialist Palliative Care Services London; 2003.
3 Leng G. A year of acupuncture in palliative care. *Palliat Med* 1999; 13: 163–4.
4 Johnstone PAS, Polston GR, Nieimtzow R *et al*. Integration of acupuncture into the oncology clinic. *Palliat Med* 2002; 16: 235–9.
5 Shen J, Wenger N, Glaspy J *et al*. Electro-acupuncture for control of myeloablative chemotherapy-induced emesis: a randomized controlled trial. *JAMA* 2000; 284: 2755–61.
6 Filshie J, Penn K, Ashley S *et al*. Acupuncture for the relief of cancer-related breathlessness. *Palliat Med* 1996; 10: 145–50.
7 Blom M, Davidson I, Fernberg J *et al*. Acupuncture treatment of patients with radiation-induced xerostomia. *Eur J Cancer B Oral Oncol* 1996; 32B: 182–90.

8   Wyon Y, Lindgren R, Hammar M *et al*. Acupuncture against climacteric disorders? Lower number of symptoms after menopause. *Lakartidningen* 1994; 91: 2318–22.

9   Yan L. Treatment of persistent hiccupping with electro-acupuncture at 'hiccup-relieving' point. *J Tradit Chin Med* 1988; 8: 23–30.

10 Grossarth-Maticek R, Kiene H, Baumgartner SM *et al*. Use of Iscador and extract of European mistletoe (Viscum album), in cancer treatment: prospective non-randomized and randomized matched pair studies nested within a cohort study. *Altern Ther* 2001; 7: 57–75.

11 Kirsch I, Montgomery G and Sapirstein G. Hypnosis as an adjunct to cognitive-behavioural psychotherapy, a meta-analysis. *J Consult Clin Psychol* 1995; 63: 214–20.

12 Benjenke CJ. Benefits of early interventions with cancer patients: a clinician's 15 year observations. *Hypnosis* 2000; 27: 75–81.

13 Lynn SJ, Kirsch I, Barabasy A *et al*. Hypnosis as an empirically supported clinical intervention: The state of the evidence and a look to the future. *Int J Clin Exp Hypn* 2000; 48: 239–59.

14 Kreiger D. *Research Backs Therapeutic Touch*. Bristol: Bristol Press; 1993.

15 Kreiger D. *Living the Therapeutic Touch: healing as a lifestyle*. New York: Dodd Mead and Co; 1987.

Further reading

- Mackereth P, Carter A, editors. *Massage and Bodywork: adapting therapies for cancer care*. London: Churchill Livingstone; 2006.

Contacts

- *National Council for Hospice and Specialist Palliative Care Services*: www.hospice-spc-council.org.uk; 1st floor, 34–44 Britannia Street, London WC1X 9JG; tel: 020 7520 8299
- *Macmillan Cancer Support*: www.macmillan.org.uk; 89 Albert Embankment, London SE1 7UQ; tel: 020 7840 7840

Evaluation and evidence-based medicine

30

Setting up an integrated health service

Change takes but an instant.
It is resistance to change that can take a lifetime.

Old Hebrew proverb

In our own practice at Huntley Mount Medical Centre, Bury, Greater Manchester, we decided to explore the possibilities of extending the provision of complementary services.

As a two-doctor practice, one partner is a homeopath. A fully integrated approach for homeopathy was already established alongside an in-house counselling service, providing a holistic and integrated approach to our patients' care. Our medical centre is based in the heart of a deprived area, and around 60% of our patients live in the poorest section of the community. We have the full spectrum of social class, most professions are represented and living in the more affluent parts of the town. We wanted to offer a wider range of complementary therapies to enhance our existing set-up to improve healthcare provision for our local community.

With careful planning the following decisions were made by the practice:

- *funding* was granted from the single regeneration budget (SRB) for three years
- *meetings* were organised of interested stakeholders with the SRB board, Barbara Heron our lead therapist, doctors and the practice manager. A joint bid, to provide six complementary therapies in-house from our practice was successful. The service was open to all 5000 residents of East Ward, irrespective of whether they were registered with our practice or not
- the *therapies chosen* were based on need and availability of therapists, and were: **aromatherapy, hypnotherapy, massage, reflexology, Reiki and shiatsu**
- *number of sessions*: one session of each therapy a week was provided so that there would be six 3-hour sessions per week
- *a dedicated room* was provided for complementary therapies in the quietest part of the building
- *fees* for the therapists were determined from the available budget for each treatment session. If a patient did not attend a session, then only half the rate was paid
- each patient was eligible for a *maximum of 10 sessions*
- all patients' *referrals* were communicated by letter; a therapist was responsible for assessing, allocating and sending appointments to patients
- doctors, practice nurses and counsellors only were *permitted to refer patients* to the scheme. Self-referrals were not allowed
- the medical conditions focused on for treatment were: **back pain, arthritis, stress, anxiety, depression, diabetes mellitus**
- any *clinical problems* would be dealt with by verbal discussion between the therapist and the doctor

- *discharge letters* were sent on completion of the course of treatment
- *evaluation* using Measure Yourself Medical Outcome Profile (MYMOP) was conducted during and on completion of the therapy (*see* Chapter 31)
- *an information pack* was compiled for patients and the other practices in the locality with access to the service
- *teamwork*: comprehensive initial planning ensured a smooth-running scheme for referring, which provided a holistic care model for patients
- *a clinical audit* is detailed in Chapter 33
- a regular *newsletter* from the team kept the participating practices in the area informed.

In setting up a service a practice team could employ one or two therapists initially. After gaining experience and confidence, further therapies could be added according to practice needs. Doctors and nurses may also decide to train and gain experience in a particular therapy as part of their professional development programme.

Practice-based commissioning (PBC) is now a realistic option providing long-term funding.

Doctors referring to complementary therapists

Doctors referring to other medics who are trained in a complementary therapy, for example acupuncture, hypnotherapy or homeopathy, have no additional ethical problem. The complementary medical practitioner assumes responsibility for medical care given.

The Medical Act of 1858 made the provision for unconventional medical treatments to be used by doctors as long as professional standards of care are adhered to. The 'Bolam test' is used to establish whether these standards of care have been met.[1]

A practice employing therapists who are not medically qualified needs to consider the following guidelines to avoid medicolegal problems:

- *professional status*: the therapist must be a member of a professional body
- *indemnity insurance cover*
- *qualifications and experience* need to be confirmed
- *an annual check of documentation* should be conducted to ensure that it is up to date
- *self-employed status* of many therapists needs to be considered.

The Prince's Foundation for Integrated Health

The Prince's Foundation was set up to enable the setting of standards of complementary care and to set the agenda for the development of therapies within the NHS for equity.[2–4]

Key principles of the Prince's Foundation for Integrated Health

- Promoting a **holistic and integrated approach to health care**
- Emphasising key principle of **individuals taking more responsibility**

- Acknowledging the **intrinsic healing capacity** of every person and awareness that different approaches and interventions may need to be employed together to restore health and 'wellbeing'
- Establishing an **evidence base** for integrated health
- Accepting that every patient should have access to the **treatment approach of their choice**
- Accepting that patients have a right to expect healthcare services to be provided by **appropriately educated, safe, competent and regulated practitioners.**

The foundation provides practitioner guidance for training and development in complementary and integrated health care. An online directory of courses is available. Support is provided with practical tools for setting up and managing an integrated health service, including sample contracts, pro forma templates and example business cases for commissioning bodies. The foundation is an invaluable resource centre.

> *All humanity is one undivided and indivisible family.*
> *Mahatma Gandhi[5]*

References

1 *Bolam v. Friern.* HMC(1957) 2 All ER 118.
2 The Prince's Foundation for Integrated Health. *Complementary Medicine Information Pack for Primary Care Groups.* London, The Prince's Foundation for Integrated Health; 2000.
3 Thomson A. *A Healthy Partnership, Integrating Complementary Healthcare into Primary Care.* London: The Prince's Foundation for Integrated Health; 2005.
4 The Prince's Foundation for Integrated Health. *Setting the Agenda for the Future.* London: The Prince's Foundation for Integrated Health; 2003.
5 Gandhi M. *The Collected Works of Mahatma Gandhi.* New Delhi: Publications Division, Government of India; 1982.

Contacts

For training courses, research, accreditation of therapists and further information on integrated health care:

- *The National Library for Health, Complementary and Alternative Medicine Specialist Library*: www.library.nhs.uk/cam
- *The Prince's Foundation for Integrated Health*: www.fih.org.uk; 33–41 Dallington Street, London EC1V 0BQ; tel: 020 3119 3100; fax 020 3119 3101

31

Evaluation

Measure Yourself Medical Outcome Profile (MYMOP)

This is a patient-centred assessment of the outcome of treatment. The patients' interpretation, progress and priorities in their clinical symptoms are used to measure the outcome of treatment with complementary therapies. The MYMOP can also be used in measuring the outcome of conventional medicine.[1] This is a useful tool well suited to primary care evaluations. When a multidisciplinary team is involved it is helpful to demonstrate effectiveness in their clinical work.

Advantages of MYMOP

- The patient decides which symptoms to measure because those symptoms are deemed to be the most important for the patient in their illness.
- The patient chooses the score variables.
- MYMOP gives a realistic sensitive measure of illness over a given period of time.
- It can be applied to the whole primary care spectrum of illness seen.
- It is capable of measuring a wide range of symptoms whether they are conventional or complementary.
- MYMOP is simple and brief, and it is possible for most patients to complete it within 10 minutes.

Studies have demonstrated that involving the patient in the outcome measurement is highly responsive to change over time, while still remaining brief in its application.[1]

Methodology for MYMOP

The MYMOP has four scales:

- the first two scales are for two symptoms that the patient chooses as being the most important
- the third scale is for an activity in daily living which has been disrupted or prevented by the illness and which the patient specifies
- the fourth scale is a rating on general feeling of 'wellbeing'.

All ratings are for the previous week, and a score on a scale of 1–7 is circled; 1 is as good as it could be and 7 as bad as it could be. On second and subsequent profiles the wording of the questionnaire is the same, but an optional fifth item for a new symptom is included. The profile score is calculated as the mean of the scored items.

In our own study at Huntley Mount Medical Centre, 47 patients were involved during part of the ongoing study illustrating the MYMOP progress of this group of patients. The graph in Figure 31.1 illustrates the mapping of the individual score change for each patient, and at the same time gives a visual analogue scale, which shows the progress achieved. As a multidisciplinary team we were able to appreciate the levels of care benefiting our patients.

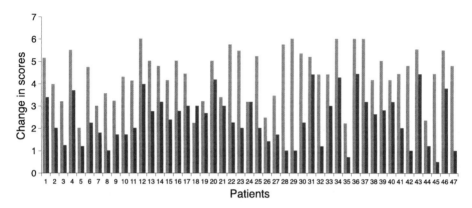

Figure 31.1   Changes in scores for MYMOP.

Audit of outcome study

Another method of measuring our work is for a simple clinical audit, which could be conducted by keeping a log. The Glasgow Homeopathic Hospital Outcome Scale (GHHOS) is one example of this method of data collection and analysis.[2,3]

Workload implications for primary care

At our medical centre we have demonstrated the reduction in workload for doctors from patients who received complementary therapy and treatments (*see* Chapter 33).

Our practice workload for GP (face-to-face) consultations over the years has been gradually reduced to 2 (compared to an average of 5 in the UK [the consultation rate is calculated by dividing the total number of consultations over a 1-year period by the number of patients on a doctor's list]).[4]

This was achieved by a **10-point plan**:

1 *continuity of care* by maintaining personal lists
2 *integration* of complementary therapies to enable patient self-care and responsibility for their illness
3 *a holistic approach* in all aspects of care including social aspects of an illness
4 *delegating* to the multidisciplinary team where appropriate
5 *educating* frequent attendees
6 *explanation and reassurance* by dealing with all symptoms and worries presented by patients, avoiding further anxiety

7 *telephone consultations* for results of investigations. Many laboratory reports can be discussed at designated times by telephone, reassurance can then be given, a referral made, or a follow-up arranged with the doctor or nurse as appropriate
8 emphasising *prevention, a healthier lifestyle and reinforcing responsibility for self-care*
9 *proactive care with opportunistic screening*
10 *easy access* to clinicians, good communication skills and team work.

> *The mathematical sciences particularly exhibit order, symmetry and limitation; and these are the greatest forms of the beautiful.*
>
> *Aristotle*

References

1 Patterson C. Measuring outcomes in primary care: a patient generated measure, MYMOP, compared with the SF-36 health survey. *BMJ* 1996; 312: 1016–20.
2 Sevar R. Audit of outcome in 455 consecutive patients treated with homeopathic medicines. *Homeopathy* 2005; 94: 215–21.
3 Robinson T. Responses to homeopathic treatment in National Health Service general practice. *Homeopathy* 2006; 95: 9–14.
4 Office of Health Economics. *Compendium of Health Statistics* (15e). London: Office of Health Economics; 2004.

Further reading

- Peters D, Chaitow L, Harris G *et al. Integrating Complementary Therapies in Primary Care.* London: Churchill Livingstone; 2002.
- White C. Reprot: *Developing Clinical Governance for Complementary and Alternative Medicine in Primary Care* 4 seminars, School of Integrated Health, University of Westminster. London: King's Fund; 2003. www.wmin.ac.uk/sih (accessed 17 October 2006).

32

The evidence for complementary therapies

The weight of evidence we have examined suggests that complementary and alternative medicine could play a much larger role in the delivery of health care, and help to fill recognised effectiveness gaps in health care provision. Illnesses such as anxiety, stress and depression and a number of chronic complaints can often be more effectively dealt with by complementary therapies.

In conclusion; Complementary Medicine remains out of reach for many low income families, those who we have found would most benefit from its provision. We believe there is a strong case for Health Ministers to recommend that the National Institute for Health and Clinical Excellence (NICE) carry out a full clinical assessment of the cost-effectiveness of such therapies.

Christopher Smallwood[1]

Assessment and evaluation are important modern-day clinical tools. The involvement of NICE would be welcomed, leading to a natural progression and development of integrated health care by evidence-based medicine.

Some encouraging statistics

- 75% of patients in a recent survey wish to see complementary medicine available within the NHS (see www.internethealthlibrary.com/surveys/surveys-uk-comp-therapies-nhs.htm).
- 50% of primary care practices provide access to complementary medicine.
- 43% of primary care trusts fund complementary therapies.
- 10% of the population uses complementary therapies at any one time.
- 30% of the population in the UK access complementary medicine, many privately; equity of access, therefore, means it should be provided by the NHS.
- Worldwide, there is widespread use of complementary medicine.[2–4] Access by the population in:
  - USA is 50%
  - Australia is 57%
  - Germany is 46%
  - France is 49%.
- Around 80% of patients using complementary medicine in the UK are satisfied with the treatment they received.[5]

The effectiveness gaps in healthcare provision

Effectiveness gaps left by conventional medicine and served more effectively by complementary medicine are particularly suited to integration. The following conditions emerge well for evidence of efficacy:

- back pain
- musculoskeletal problems
- arthritis
- depression
- anxiety
- stress
- chronic pain management
- asthma
- migraine
- palliative care.

Cost-effectiveness

Many therapies pay for themselves in the longer term. Our own study in 'An investigation into the impact of integrating complementary and alternative medicine into conventional general practice' has studied this (*see* Chapter 33).

The Smallwood report concludes and recommends the following:[1]

- a number of complementary therapies offer the possibility of significant savings in direct health costs
- some therapies, just as expensive as their conventional counterparts, can nonetheless deliver additional benefits to patients in a cost-effective way
- the benefits to the economy of a wider application of successful complementary therapies could run into hundreds of millions of pounds
- evidence from the literature review indicates that many of the main complementary therapies are effective and can contribute to the effectiveness gap in NHS care
- NICE could conduct a full assessment of cost-effectiveness and effectiveness of the therapies for the potential role within the NHS
- in deprived areas, where communities are denied the benefits of complementary therapies, NHS savings in the long-term chronic care of patients could take place. There is strong evidence to give priority to deprived areas. (Our own outcome study (*see* Chapter 33) was conducted on patients from a deprived area in Bury, Greater Manchester. This research evidence supports the Smallwood report's recommendation on making complementary therapies available to the populations of deprived areas within the umbrella of the NHS. Our practice found that for the study group, a 30% reduction in consultation rate took place for the year following completion of a therapy)
- primary care should continue the 'gatekeeper' role for the NHS and provision of complementary therapies, and then can become a truly integrated healthcare service. Conflict between conventional and complementary therapies will, therefore, be minimised

- practice-based commissioning (PBC) is a source of funding for complementary therapies, and primary care can then develop the necessary services to meet all the health needs of the population
- regional differences in provision of complementary therapies need to be balanced. London has a much greater provision
- funding for research should be increased substantially from its current 0.08% of the NHS research budget and 0.3% of the research budget of UK charities
- complementary therapy research organisations should collaborate in order to develop a unified research programme, so as to establish a rigorous evidence base relating not only to costs but also to the benefits of complementary therapies for the future.

Organisations facilitating integration of complementary medicine

- The Prince's Foundation of Integrated Health supported by the King's Fund
- The World Health Organization (WHO)
- The National Centre for Complementary and Alternative Medicine (NCCAM) USA
- The Centre for Complementary Medicine Research, University of Western Sydney, Sydney, Australia
- The Office of Cancer Complementary and Alternative Medicine (OCCAM)

There are seven complementary medicine centres of excellence worldwide. These are defined as having researchers with more than 20 MEDLINE publications. Three of these are in the USA, two in the UK and one each in Germany and Switzerland.[6]

Research methodology

Life is never straightforward, and neither is conventional research methodology applied to complementary medicine. Nevertheless, it is very important to apply reproducible research techniques to validate the effectiveness of the complementary therapies applied to human patients and, to a certain extent, animals.

Research needs to supply answers to questions about:

- effectiveness
- safety
- cost-effectiveness
- comparison to conventional treatment models
- evaluation:
  - against placebo
  - with conventional treatment
  - quality assurance.

There are difficulties in the methodology of undertaking complementary medicine research which need to be acknowledged, accepted and taken into account.[6] The majority of complementary therapies involve a crucial and essential interaction between the patient and the practitioner. This, therefore, makes it difficult to create a suitable placebo. Therapies are often tailored to individual needs. Homeopathy, in particular, and many of the other alternative treatments are based on a different diagnostic process from conventional medicine. Often homeopathy and Reiki are used together. Similarly in traditional Chinese medicine, not only is acupuncture used, but dietary and lifestyle advice are given together with herbal remedies. It is therefore difficult in this instance to 'fragment' the holism and study each component separately. This synergistic effect with the complementary therapies needs further research.

To compound the difficulties even more, consider the following study.

Case study 32.1

An orthopaedic surgeon decided to conduct a controlled trial of arthroscopic surgery for osteoarthritis of the knee. Five patients were given the real surgery and five were given only a small incision over the knee to make it appear that they had arthroscopic surgery. Patients were followed up for two years. The pain and swelling were reduced in the majority of the placebo group as well as in the patients that received the real surgery. A follow-up trial of 180 patients confirmed the same results.[7]

This illustrates the value of placebo-controlled trials in determining the efficacy of drugs and of medical procedures.

Types of research study

Double-blind trial

A double-blind trial is particularly difficult in complementary therapy research, because of the many factors involved in holistic care. Patients may be able to discern whether they are receiving the 'real' treatment or the placebo. A person may detect the 'real' treatment because of the smell or taste of a liquid preparation. Preparing a substance that looks and tastes similar to a placebo treatment is difficult. This means that the patients in the treatment group would know they are taking the real substance and those in the placebo group would know they are taking placebo. This effectively invalidates the whole trial. Similarly when patients take the 'real' substance in a trial where the treatment produces side-effects this makes the patient and the researchers aware that those patients were on the 'real' substance or treatment.

It is therefore challenging for researchers to design a double-blind placebo-controlled trial in acupuncture, diet, surgery, Reiki, massage, reflexology, aromatherapy, osteopathy or chiropractic. Even in 'well-designed' double-blind studies, unexpected difficulties arise, for example the participants may not be a representative sample of the general population being studied.

The statistical analysis of any trial is important in analysing the results. The size of the study is always significant. If, for example, the treatment of depression is being studied, a large number of patients are required to enable significant results to be meaningful scientifically and demonstrate benefit. In antidepressant studies where patients are given placebo, about 75% report an improvement, as much as in the treated group. The other factor in this type of study is that questionnaires for depression scales are open to wide variations of interpretation. To overcome this, large trials are designed for meaningful data to be obtained. Small trials in homeopathy or herbal medicine for example, that do not prove efficacy, do not mean the remedies do not work. Larger trials need to be conducted.

If too many outcomes are measured in any trial, by chance alone some indicators may show an improvement. Therefore, to eliminate this only the original planned primary outcome measures are valid.

Double-blind comparative trial

A double-blind comparative trial involves comparing a new treatment against an established one. If the new treatment is equally effective, then such a study gives proof of effectiveness. A placebo group, however, should be used to give more meaningful results.

Single-blind study

In this type of study, the researchers are aware of who is receiving the real treatment, and the patients that are not. Acupuncture, surgery, massage and chiropractic studies are usually single-blind trials.

Single-blind trials cannot, therefore, eliminate the placebo effect. In acupuncture, for instance, the therapist knows which patients received the treatment, and another researcher, who does not know which patients received the designated treatment, evaluates the outcome.

Controlled study using an untreated group

A proportion of the patients who do not receive the treatment are compared to the treatment group. This poses all the problems so far discussed.

Observational study

Also known as intervention trials, many of these have been conducted in complementary medicine and particularly in homeopathy. Large groups are studied for meaningful results. A six-year study involving homeopathic treatment of chronic diseases in Bristol concluded:

> *homeopathic intervention offered positive health changes to a substantial proportion of a large cohort (6544) of patients with a wide range of chronic diseases. Additional observational research, including studies using different designs, is necessary for further research development in homeopathy.*[8]

Observational studies are often the only practical way to gain an understanding about long-term health problems, such as nutrition and lifestyle, that are not amenable to placebo. Many such studies therefore involve a follow-up of patients for decades, in order to obtain valued data. It is not possible to conduct double-blind studies under such conditions to meet the requirements necessary for a truly double-blind placebo-controlled trial.

In vitro study

Studies *in vitro* may confirm a theoretical effect of a substance and may also trigger a study to evaluate effectiveness in animals first, before trials are conducted in humans.

Of particular interest to homeopathy are the experiments that were first conducted by Professor Benaviste in 1981.[9] His experiments have been replicated successfully since, in a number of laboratories. The authors from these laboratory experiments reported that the action of high dilutions involves an effect of the solvent (water) on histamine H_2 receptors, even though it is paradoxical in terms of molecular biology, when in theory there are no molecules in the active dilutions tested. Furthermore, the high dilution was not the only factor, but there was evidence that it was the succussion (shaking process) and dilution to produce the active homeopathic remedy that produced the results reported.[9–11]

The aim of the laboratory researchers was not to justify the clinical use of homeopathic medicines but to present scientific evidence showing that the substances prepared according to the homeopathic method had some effects on the immune system and on inflammation. These findings may be the first step for a re-evaluation of homeopathy as a worthwhile field of basic clinical investigation.

Immunology and allergic reactions can represent a bridge between homeopathy and conventional medicine to facilitate a better understanding of the 'similarity' or 'similars' principle and acknowledge the great sensitivity of living systems to modulations induced by high dilutions of natural or endogenous substances (*see* Chapter 12).[12]

In all sections of the book, we have highlighted only some of the evidence available on the clinical effectiveness of the mainstream complementary therapies.

> *Some patients, though conscious that their condition is perilous, recover their health simply to their contentment of the goodness of the Physician.*
>
> *Hippocrates*

References

1 Smallwood C. *The Role of Complementary and Alternative Medicine in the NHS*. London: Fresh Minds; 2005.
2 Eisenberg DM, Davis RB, Ettner SL *et al*. Trends in alternative medicinal use in the United States, 1990–1997. *JAMA* 1998; 280:1569–75.
3 Bensoussan A. Complementary medicine – where lies its appeal? (editorial) *Med J Aust* 1999; 170: 247–8.
4 Fisher P and Ward A. Complementary medicine in Europe. *BMJ* 1994; 309:107–11.
5 Zollman C and Vickers A. Complementary medicine and the patient. *BMJ* 1999; 319: 1486–9.
6 Bensoussan A and Lewith GT. Complementary medicine research in Australia: a strategy. *Med J Aust* 2004; 181: 331–3.
7 Mosely JB, O'Malley K, Petersen NJ *et al*. A controlled trial of arthroscopic surgery for osteoarthritis of the knee. *N Engl J Med* 2002; 347: 81–8.
8 Spence DS, Thompson EA and Barron SJ. Homeopathic treatment for chronic disease: a 6-year, university-hospital outpatient observational study. *J Altern Complement Med* 2005; 11: 793–8.
9 Benaviste J. The human basophil degranulation test as an in vitro method for the diagnosis of allergies. *Clin Allergy* 1981; 11: 1–11.

10 Bellavite P, Conforti A, Pontarollo F et al. Immunology and homeopathy. 2 Cells of the immune system and inflammation. *Evid Based Complement Alternat Med* 2005; 3: 13–24.
11 Tschulakow AV Yan Y and Klimek W. A new approach to the memory of water. *Homeopathy* 2005; 94: 241–7.
12 Bellavite P, Conforti A, Piasere V et al. Immunology and homeopathy. 1 Historical background. *Evid Based Complement Alternat Med* 2005; 2: 441–52.

Contacts

- *Centre for Complementary Medicine Research, University of Western Sydney, Australia*: www.ccr.edu.au
- *National Centre for Complementary and Alternative Medicine (NCCAM) USA*: www.nccam.nih.gov
- *Office of Cancer Complementary and Alternative Medicine (OCCAM)*: www.cancer.gov/cam
- *The Prince's Foundation for Integrated Health*: www.fih.org.uk
- *World Health Organization (WHO)*: www.who.int/en

33

An investigation into the impact of integrating complementary and alternative medicine into conventional general practice

L Demetriou, B Heron** and A Demetriou*

*L Demetriou BSc (Hons), Research Assistant
**B Heron BA, PGCE, Dip SEN, Dip Aromatherapy, Advanced Massage Practitioner/Project Co-ordinator

You can't solve a problem with the same mind that created it.

Wayne Dyer[1]

Introduction

A three-year funded project for complementary and alternative medicine (CAM) was set up in 2001, based in a general practice setting. This was funded from the single regeneration budget (SRB), which was non-recurring.

Huntley Mount Medical Centre (HMMC) is a two-partner practice of 3600 patients already providing homeopathy as part of general medical services (GMS) by the senior partner. Adding six CAM therapies, aromatherapy, hypnotherapy, reflexology, Reiki, remedial massage and Shiatsu, gave the opportunity to widen the scope of integration of health care. Sixty per cent of patients of HMMC live in a deprived area and only these patients qualified for the CAM scheme, due to the funding criteria.

Methods

A half-day session of each of the six therapies was provided each week. Patients underwent up to 10 one-hour treatment sessions of the allocated therapy. In this study, data from 61 patients were collected and analysed. All of the patients studied have undergone a form of complementary therapy in the first 2 years of the project. In order to assess the impact of introducing such a scheme, a variety of data from each of these patient's records were collected and analysed. With a view to assessing the overall benefits of the scheme, comparisons were made between data sets before and after CAM. The study concentrated on the impact on cost savings and the doctor consultation rate, to assess the long-term benefits to patients.

Results

Data from 61 patients (48 females, 13 males) who underwent some form of CAM were collected.

Consultations

The number of consultations with a doctor before and after the commencement of CAM was analysed. The number of consultations each patient had with a doctor in the one year prior to introducing CAM was collected, as was the number of consultations each patient had with a doctor in the year following commencement of the therapy. Results are shown in Table 33.1 and Figure 33.1.

Table 33.1 The percentage changes in the numbers of consultations with a doctor in the year after CAM

Change	Male (%)	Female (%)	Total (%)
Decrease	69	71	71
Same	8	8	8
Increase	23	21	21

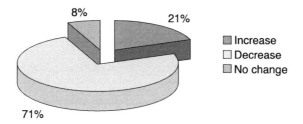

Figure 33.1 Graph of the percentage change in the number of consultations with a doctor following CAM.

As can be seen in Figure 33.1, the majority of patients exhibited a decrease in the number of visits to a doctor in the one year following commencement of a CAM. However, the statistical significance of this must be determined.

Statistical analysis

The data were checked to see if they were normally distributed and to get descriptive statistics.

For consultations before CAM

- Mean = 8.49 ± 0.83 SE (standard error)
- K/S (Kolmogorov–Smirnov) test for normality
- Result: Stat = 0.147, df (degrees of freedom) = 61, $P = 0.002$
- **Data are significant and therefore not normally distributed.**

For consultations after CAM

- Mean = 5.9 ± 0.60 SE
- K/S test for normality
- Result: Stat = 0.164, df (degrees of freedom) = 61, $P < 0.001$
- **Data are significant and therefore not normally distributed.**

Results of the Wilcoxon signed ranks test gave this output:

- $Z = -4.254$
- $n = 61$
- $P < 0.001$

This is a significant result, hence there is a significant difference between the number of consultations before and after therapy – this significant difference is in fact a significant decrease.

The large percentage of male and female patients who exhibited a decrease in their number of consultations with a doctor after the therapy can be seen in Figure 33.2. The combined total number of consultations attended by the 61 patients in the one year before and in the year following commencement of CAM can be seen in Table 33.2. This table demonstrates an overall 30.5% reduction in consultations following CAM.

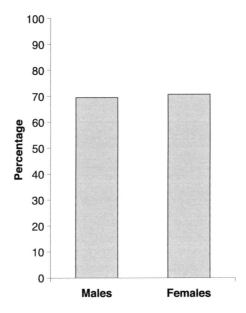

Figure 33.2 Bar chart showing the percentage of male/female patients treated with CAM exhibiting a subsequent decrease in numbers of consultations with a doctor.

Table 33.2   Total number of consultations and percentage reduction following CAM

	Total number of consultations
Before CAM	518
After CAM	360
Difference	158
% Change	−30.5%

Prescribing

The number of prescriptions issued to each patient in the one year period prior to commencement of CAM was compared with the number issued in the one year following CAM therapy. Results are shown in Tables 33.3 and 33.4 and Figure 33.3.

Table 33.3   The total number of prescriptions issued and percentage change before and after CAM

	Total number of prescriptions
Before CAM	1713
After CAM	1809
Difference	96
% Change	+5.6%

Table 33.4   The percentage changes in number of prescriptions issued following CAM

Change	Male (%)	Female (%)	Total (%)
Decrease	54	42	44
Same	8	6	7
Increase	38	52	49

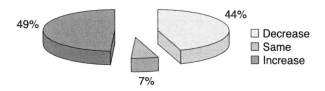

Figure 33.3   Graph of the percentage change in number of prescriptions issued following CAM.

In order to establish whether these results were significant, i.e. whether there had been a significant increase or decrease in the number of prescriptions issued to patients after CAM, further statistical analysis was required.

Statistical analysis

First the data were checked to see if they were normally distributed and to get descriptive statistics.

For prescriptions 1 year before CAM

- Mean (of the data set) = 28.08 ± 3.683 (standard error, SE)
- Since $n = 61$, the Kolmogorov–Smirnov test (K/S test) was used to test to see whether the data were normally distributed.
- Result: Stat = 0.173; degrees of freedom (df) = 61; $P < 0.001$.
- This is a significant result, and means the **data are not normally distributed**.

For prescriptions 1 year after CAM

- Mean = 29.66 ± 3.912 SE
- K/S test for normality
- Result: Stat = 0.168, df = 61, $P < 0.001$
- **Data are not normally distributed.**

Since both sets of data are from the same people and they are both non-normal, we used the Wilcoxon signed ranks test, the non-parametric version of the paired samples t test.

Results of the Wilcoxon signed ranks test gave this output:

- $Z = -0.942$
- $n = 61$
- $P = 0.346$.

This P value indicates a non-significant result. From this we can say that there is no significant difference between the two sets of data – hence there has been no significant change in the number of prescriptions issued following CAM.

Discussion

Consultations

For the one year following CAM therapy, a 30% reduction in consultation rate was achieved for the 61 patients (*see* Table 33.2). This translates to 158 consultations, which at locum rates saves £2700 in doctor time. If all 77 patients who underwent CAM achieved the same result this would equate to a £3600 saving in doctor consultation time. The 16 patients not included in the study belonged to other medical centres and data were not available for the study. Only patients registered at HMMC were included in the data collected. Doctor access can therefore be improved significantly by use of CAM.

Prescribing

As shown by the output of the Wilcoxon statistical test, total prescribing for all patients collectively did not show a significant difference in the year following CAM therapy. However 44% of patients did show a reduction in prescribing, and a further 7% exhibited no increase in prescriptions following CAM (*see* Figure 33.3). This left 49% of patients who did show some increase in prescriptions. This however could be attributable to the fact that a significant number of patients were encouraged by the CAM to go on to smoking cessation and resolving other health issues. Over a longer period, an overall reduction in prescribing may well be achieved; however this is a separate study, which may be conducted on this group of patients in the future.

Implications for the future

HMMC had a prescribing budget of £530 000 for the financial year ending March 2003. A £113 000 prescribing saving was made (21%) due to the holistic approach. The opportunity to make this saving was initiated when a partner (not trained in complementary therapies) retired from the practice and the homeopath/GP took over the overall prescribing and prudence for the whole practice. This prescribing saving relates to the list of 3600 patients overall. A separate analysis for the patients in the study shows a more complicated picture. However, we are convinced that the savings from prescribing and using CAM can be made to pay for the complementary therapy scheme. Some insight into logistical approaches to quality, equality and rational use of funding can create a more widespread NHS use of CAM. A longer study, probably over 5 years, may show even more benefits, making out a good case for financing and supporting CAM in the NHS.

> *The soul manifests in the world in order that it may experience the different phases of manifestation yet not lose its way, but regain its original freedom in addition to the experience and knowledge it has gleaned in the world.*
>   *Hazrat Inayat Khan*[2]

References

1 Dyer W. *10 Secrets for Success and Inner Peace*. London: Hay House; 2005.
2 Khan PZI (ed). *A Pearl in Wine: Essays in the Life, Music and Sufism of Hazrat Inayat Khan*. New Lebanon, NY: Omega; 2001.

Index

abuse 8, 54, 58
acne 62, 140–1
Aconite napellis (Monkshood)
   anxiety 8, 11
   death and dying 34, 38
   ear, nose and throat 147, 148, 151, 152, 169,
     170
   paediatric medicine 169, 170
   stress 19
   symptom complex 72
Actea racemosa 64
acupressure 147
acupuncture
   chronic disease 126–8, 131, 134, 135
   dermatology 141, 142
   ear, nose and throat 146, 148, 149, 150
   headaches 156, 157
   obstetrics and gynaecology 158, 159, 160, 161
   overview 45–8
   paediatric medicine 171
   palliative care 175
   research studies 182, 190, 191
   traditional Chinese medicine 108, 109
addiction 22, 23, 58, 80, 109, 116
additives 118, 139, 171
adrenaline 8, 10, 15, 87, 88
Aesculus 127
Agaricus 131
Age Concern 42
Age-Related Eye Disease Study 133
aggravations 71, 72, 74, 143
Agnus castus 62, 64, 160, 164
Ailanthus 153
alcohol
   anxiety 8
   Ayurvedic medicine 54
   bereavement 39
   coronary heart disease 137
   depression 22, 23, 27
   eczema 142
   essential hypertension 135
   health and lifestyle 115, 116, 117
   Islam 30–1
   menopause 165
   stress 15
Alexander technique 93, 129
Alfalfa 164
allergies
   asthma 134, 170
   health and lifestyle 117–18, 122
   research studies 192
   stress 16
   traditional Chinese medicine 109
   urticaria 139
Allium cepa 149, 152
Allium sativa see garlic
Aloe vera 55, 62, 64–5, 127
alternative medicine see complementary and
    alternative medicine

American Medical Association (AMA)
   79
American Psychiatric Association 79
anaemia 22, 116
anaesthesia 79, 80
analgesics 46, 62, 95, 101, 115
anger
   anxiety 8
   bereavement 37, 38
   depression 21, 24, 27
   homeopathy 71, 75
   massage 83
   stress 17, 18
anorexia nervosa 8, 12, 116
antenatal care 158–9
antibiotics
   acne 140
   cystitis 162
   health and lifestyle 115, 117
   homeopathy 70
   integrated health care 2
   paediatric medicine 167
   sinusitis 151
antidepressants 24, 25, 62, 65, 115, 190–1
Antimonium crudum 141
Antimonium tartaricum 135, 140, 169
anxiety 7–14
   acupuncture 175
   aromatherapy 49, 50, 51
   asthma 134
   contacts 14
   counselling 58
   death and dying 29, 33
   depression 22
   diabetes mellitus 133
   essential hypertension 136
   evidence-based medicine 181, 187, 188
   health and lifestyle 116, 118
   herbal medicine 62, 65
   homeopathy 18, 71–5, 175, 176
   hypnotherapy 176
   management 8–10
   massage 83, 84, 85, 86
   meditation 88
   obsessive–compulsive behaviour 11–13
   overview 7–8
   palliative care 175, 176, 177
   panic attacks 10–11
   prayer 97, 98
   reflexology 102
   Reiki healing 106
   stress 15, 17, 18, 19
   yoga 113
Apis mellifica 139, 158, 169
Aquinas, Thomas 15
Arbor vitae see Thuja
Argentum nitricum (silver nitrate) 8, 71–2, 126,
    133, 136, 159
Aristotle 186

Arnica montana (Leopard's bane)
  antenatal care 158
  anxiety 9
  backache 129
  death and dying 34, 38
  headaches 156, 157
  homeopathic treatment 72, 73
  influenza 153
  leg cramps 130
aromatherapy
  chronic disease 127, 130, 131, 134, 135
  death and dying 34
  dermatology 140–1, 142, 144
  ear, nose and throat 147, 149, 150
  evidence-based medicine 181, 190, 194
  herbal medicine 61, 62
  history, philosophy and evidence 49–50
  obstetrics and gynaecology 161, 165
  overview 49–52
  palliative care 177
Arsenicum album (white oxide of arsenic)
  antenatal care 158
  anxiety 8, 12
  asthma 135, 170
  cardiology 134
  death and dying 34
  dermatology 139, 142, 143
  ear, nose and throat 149, 152
  neuralgias 131
  paediatric medicine 169, 170
  stress 18
  symptom complex 72
Arsenicum iodatum 149
arthritis
  evidence-based medicine 181, 188
  herbal medicine 63, 65
  massage 85
  nutritional medicine 116
  osteoarthritis and rheumatoid arthritis 127–8
  osteopathy and chiropractic 93, 94
  reflexology 102
ASH (Action on Smoking and Health) 20
assertiveness training 18
assisted dying 29
asthma
  children 95, 170
  chronic disease 134–5
  eczema 142
  evidence-based medicine 188
  homeopathy 73, 74, 75
  hypnotherapy 79
  massage 84
  meditation 88
  nutritional medicine 116
  osteopathy and chiropractic 93, 94, 95
  premenstrual syndrome 160
  reflexology 102
  traditional Chinese medicine 109
  yoga 113
athlete's foot 51, 63
atopy 109, 117, 134, 142, 143
attention deficit syndrome 170
attitude awareness 18
Aurum met 12, 23
autism 120, 170

Avena sativa 8, 11, 12, 18, 34, 38, 164
Avogadro's law 68
Ayurvedic medicine 53–5, 61, 92

Bach flower remedies 61
back pain
  antenatal care 159
  anxiety 7
  chronic disease 128–9
  evidence-based medicine 181, 188
  homeopathy 74
  massage 84
  osteopathy and chiropractic 92, 93, 95–6
  reflexology 102
Baird, David 68
Baryta carbonica 169
basil 130, 131, 149, 165
Bayley, Doreen 101
Beck Anxiety Inventory 12
bedwetting 170
behavioural therapy 11, 12, 59, 170, 176
Belladonna (deadly nightshade)
  ear, nose and throat 146, 148, 151, 152, 153, 169
  homeopathic treatment 69, 70
  osteoarthritis and rheumatoid arthritis 128
  paediatric medicine 168, 169
  urethral syndrome 162
Benaviste, Professor J 192
benign paroxymal positional vertigo 146–7
benign prostatic hypertrophy (BPH) 65, 136–7
bereavement
  counselling 58, 59
  death and dying 33, 35
  depression 27
  headaches 157
  homeopathy 71
  massage 86
  overview 36–42
  palliative care 174
  prayer 98
  yoga 113
bergamot 144, 150
Berger, Hans 79
Bhagavad Vita 112
bhutas (elements) 53
Billett, Professor Ellen 24
Black cohosh (Cimcifuja racemosa) 64, 164
Black snakeroot 64
blood pressure
  anxiety 9, 10
  childhood obesity 172
  depression 24
  essential hypertension 135–6
  exercise 118
  massage 85
  meditation 88
  prayer 98
  stress 19
BMA *see* British Medical Association
BMJ see British Medical Journal
Bolam test 182
bone marrow transplants 176
Borax 146, 147
Bowen technique 92, 93
BPH *see* benign prostatic hypertrophy

Bradshaw, John 7, 83
Braid, James 79
brain 15, 46, 79, 100, 121, 156
breast cancer 164, 175, 176
breast feeding 116, 118
breathing
    anxiety 10–11
    asthma 135
    death and dying 34
    massage 85
    meditation 88, 89
    palliative care 175
    relaxation 120
    stress 17
    traditional Chinese medicine 108
    yoga 112
British Medical Association (BMA) 79
British Medical Journal (BMJ) 79, 116
Brooks, David 2
Bryonia (Wild hops) 70, 127, 129, 146, 152, 164, 169
Buddhism 31–2, 35, 87, 90, 98, 120
bulimia 116
burdock 140, 143
burns 50, 51, 80
Bushmaster snake *see* Lachesis

Caesar, Julius 84
Caesarean section 158
cajuput 140
Calcarea 130, 140–3, 150, 153, 168–9
calcium
    depression 24, 26
    diet 9, 18, 117
    menopause 165
    multiple sclerosis 132
    osteoporosis 129
calendula 140, 142, 158
Calm helpline 27
CAM *see* complementary and alternative medicine
camomile 126, 127, 140, 142, 150, 159
cancer
    death and dying 28, 35
    depression 21
    massage 84, 85, 86
    menopause 164
    nutritional medicine 116, 117
    palliative care 174–8
    prayer 98
    reflexology 102
    traditional Chinese medicine 109
Cannabis indica 132
Cantharis (Spanish fly) 68, 73, 162
Capsicum 152
caraway seeds 61
Carbo vegetabilis 158, 170
cardiology 134
cataracts 65
catarrh 51, 63, 65, 75, 149–51
Catholicism 30, 40, 41
Caulophyllum 158
Causticum 131, 137, 141, 152, 162, 169
cayenne 148
cedar wood 49, 149

Centre for Complementary Medicine Research, Australia 189, 193
cerebral palsy 85, 95
cerebrovascular accident (CVA) 130
Chamomilla 71, 73, 168, 170
chaparral 142
CHD *see* coronary heart disease
chemotherapy 31, 81, 84, 109, 176, 177
chi *see* qi
chickenpox 143, 169
chickweed 140
childbirth 51, 72, 80, 86
children
    aromatherapy 49
    asthma 134, 170
    Ayurvedic medicine 55
    bereavement 35, 36, 37, 38
    death and dying 32, 33, 35
    healthy eating and lifestyle 118, 119, 171–2
    hypnotherapy 80
    massage 83
    osteopathy and chiropractic 93, 94, 95
    otitis media 148, 169
    paediatric medicine 167–73
Chinese cultural beliefs 31–2 *see also* traditional Chinese medicine
chiropractic 84, 91–6, 129, 190–1
cholesterol 64, 137
chondroitin 128
Chopra, Deepak 61
Christianity 30, 31, 39, 87, 97
chronic disease 125–38
    asthma 134–5
    backache 128–9
    benign prostatic hypertrophy 136–7
    cardiology 134
    cerebrovascular accident 130
    chronic disease management 125–6
    coronary heart disease 137
    diabetes mellitus 133
    epilepsy 136
    essential hypertension 135–6
    haemorrhoids 127
    homeopathy 71
    inflammatory bowel disease 126–7
    irritable bowel syndrome 126
    leg cramps 130
    macular degeneration 133
    multiple sclerosis 131–2
    myalgic encephalomyelitis 130
    neuralgias 131
    osteoarthritis and rheumatoid arthritis 127–8
    osteoporosis 129
    Reiki healing 106
    research studies 191
    thyroid disorders 132–3
    yoga 113
Cicely Saunders Foundation 35
Cimcifuja racemosa (Black cohosh) 64, 164
Cina 168
cinnamon 50, 55, 61, 152
circulation 45, 65, 85, 88, 109, 113
Cistus 153, 169
Citizens Advice Bureau 42
clary 165

Clematis erecta 136
client-centred therapy 56
cloves 50, 55, 131
Club moss *see* Lycopodium
cluster headaches 155, 156
Cocculus 146, 147
coffee
    anxiety 8
    bereavement 39
    eczema 142
    essential hypertension 135
    homeopathy 69
    menopause 165
    nutritional medicine 116–17
    stress 19
cognitive–behavioural therapy
        59, 176
colds 50, 51, 63, 117
colic 74, 93, 95, 126, 127, 168
Colocynth 126, 131, 168, 169
The Compassionate Friends 35, 42
complementary and alternative medicine (CAM)
    chronic disease 126
    death and dying 34
    evaluation 184–6
    in general practice 194–9
    integrated health care vi, 1–3, 181–3
    reflexology 101–2
concentration 7, 8, 65, 78, 88, 95
Conium 146
constipation 74, 75, 85, 127
constitutional remedies 18, 71, 127, 129–31, 141,
        144, 152
consultation rates 185, 186, 188, 195–7, 198
contraceptive pill 22, 55, 110, 117, 135, 160
coronary heart disease (CHD) 88, 89, 98, 118, 137
cortisol 15, 87, 89
coryza 65, 75, 169
cost-effectiveness 187, 188–9, 198, 199
coughs 50, 51, 63, 73, 155
counselling
    anxiety 7–11, 14
    bereavement 38
    death and dying 32
    depression 23, 25
    homeopathy 71
    integrated health care 181
    overview 56–60
    stress 19
crampbark 130
cramps 10, 63, 74, 85, 130, 132
cranberry juice 162
cranial osteopathy 92, 94, 168
Crataegus tincture (Hawthorn) 136
Crohn's disease *see* inflammatory bowel disease
Cruse Bereavement Care 27, 42
Cuprum metallicum 130
Curacao aloe 64
Cuttlefish ink *see* Sepia
CVA *see* cerebrovascular accident
cypress 127, 165
cystitis 63, 68, 73, 75, 162

Dalai Lama 31, 54
dandelion root 143

dandruff 51, 63
De Chardin, Pierre Teilhard 158
de Vernejoul, Pierre 46
deadly nightshade *see* Belladonna
death and dying 28–35
    aromatherapy 50
    bereavement 36–42
    complementary therapies 34
    contacts 34
    counselling 57
    cultural and religious observances
        29–32
    depression 21, 27
    dying process 32–3
    obsessive–compulsive behaviour 12
    overview 28–9
    palliative care 174–8
    prayer 97, 98
Delaney, Frank 9
Delius, Frederick 120
dementia 26, 51, 65, 116
dental care 74, 79, 95
depression
    acupuncture 175
    aromatherapy 49, 51
    cranial osteopathy 94
    diabetes mellitus 133
    evidence-based medicine 181, 187, 188, 190,
        191
    headaches 157
    herbal medicine 62, 64, 65
    homeopathy 71, 73, 74, 175, 176
    lifestyle management 116, 118
    management 23–5
    massage 83, 84, 86
    meditation 88
    multiple sclerosis 131, 132
    obsessive–compulsive behaviour
        12
    overview 21–7
    palliative care 175, 176, 177
    prayer 97, 98
    premenstrual syndrome 160
    Reiki healing 104, 105, 106
    stress 15, 16, 17
    yoga 113
dermatitis 109, 117
dermatology 139–45
    acne 140–1
    eczema 142–3
    leg ulcers 144
    psoriasis 143–4
    urticaria 139–40
    viral warts 141–2
detoxing 53, 54, 55
Devil's claw 129
diabetes mellitus 110, 116, 118, 133, 172, 181
Dickens, Charles 47
diet *see* nutritional medicine
doctors *see* GPs (general practitioners)
dopamine 24
doshas 53, 54
double-blind trials 75, 190–1
Down's syndrome 95
drug abuse 15, 22, 23, 58, 109, 116

drug interactions 55, 62, 110
Dulcamara 141, 169
duodenal ulcers 17, 74
Dyer, Wayne 1, 194
dying *see* death and dying
dysmenorrhoea 74, 75, 85, 160
dyspepsia 15, 74, 75, 116

ear, nose and throat (ENT) 146–54
    benign paroxymal positional vertigo 146–7
    catarrh 149–50
    cold sores 152
    glandular fever 153
    hay fever 148–9
    influenza 152–3
    nasal polyps 150
    osteopathy 95
    otitis media 148, 169
    reflexology 101
    sinusitis 150–1
    travel sickness 147–8
    upper respiratory tract infections 151–2
ECG *see* electrocardiogram
Echinacea 65, 140
eczema
    aromatherapy 51
    asthma 134
    depression 25
    dermatology 142–3
    homeopathy 73, 75
    nutritional medicine 116
    paediatric medicine 170
    traditional Chinese medicine 109
EEG *see* electro-encephalography
Einstein, Albert 97, 104
elderflower 150, 152, 153
elderly people
    aromatherapy 51
    Ayurvedic medicine 55
    benign prostatic hypertrophy 137
    bereavement 36, 42
    death and dying 28, 29
    depression 25–7
    hypnotherapy 81
    nutritional medicine 117
electrocardiogram (ECG) 10, 132, 134
electro-encephalography (EEG) 79
Elliotson, John 79
emotions 8, 37, 56, 57, 87, 120
empathy 18, 57, 58, 76
endogenous depression 21, 25
endorphins 46, 88, 101
ENT *see* ear, nose and throat
Epictetus 15
epilepsy 136
episiotomy 158
Epley manouvre 146–7
Equisetum 136
Esdale, James 79
essential hypertension 135–6
eucalyptus 131, 134, 149, 150
Eupatorium 152
Euphrasia 149, 169
euthanasia 29
evaluation 3, 76, 184–6

evening primrose oil 9, 51, 117, 161, 165
evidence-based medicine 179–99
    complementary therapies 187–93
    contacts 193
    cost-effectiveness 188–9
    evaluation 184–6
    in general practice 194–9
    integrated health care 2, 3, 181–3
    research methodology 189–90
    research study types 190–2
    statistics 187–8
exercise
    anxiety 8, 13
    Ayurvedic medicine 53, 54
    coronary heart disease 137
    depression 21, 24–5, 26
    essential hypertension 135
    lifestyle management 115, 118–19, 172
    multiple sclerosis 132
    obstetrics and gynaecology 161, 165
    osteopathy 95
    osteoporosis 129
    stress 18
    traditional Chinese medicine 108

fasting 30, 53, 54, 55
Feverfew 63, 65
fight or flight response 15, 87
first aid 105
Fitzgerald, Dr William 101
flatulence 74, 75, 126, 127
fluid intake 8, 39, 117, 165, 172
food *see* nutritional medicine
Food Standards Agency (FSA) 137, 171
frankincense 50, 127
Freeman, Father Laurence 121
Freud, Sigmund 49
frozen shoulder syndrome 93, 94
funerals 30, 31, 33, 40, 41, 97

Gandhi, Mahatma 53, 183
garlic (Allium sativa) 18, 55, 61, 64, 117, 150, 168
Gattefossé, René-Maurice 50
Gawain, Shakti 78
Gelsemium 8, 34, 149, 151, 152, 169
General Medical Services (GMS) 125, 194
general practitioners *see* GPs
geranium 142, 165
germander (Teucrum chamaedrys) 142
Gibran, Kahlil 34
ginger 55, 126, 130, 147, 150, 152, 159
Ginkgo biloba extracts (GBE) 65
glandular fever 22, 153, 169
Glasgow Homeopathic Hospital Outcome Scale
        (GHHOS) 185
glaucoma 65, 155
glucosamine 128
GMS *see* General Medical Services
Goethe, Johan Wolfgang von 51
GPs (general practitioners) 33, 37, 45, 185, 195–7
Graphites 142, 143, 149, 164
grief 23, 28, 31, 36–41, 73–4, 83
Gyatso, Geshe Kelsang 153
gynaecology 158–66
    antenatal care 158–9

cystitis 162
dysmenorrhoea 160
infertility 159
menopause 163–5
menorrhagia 160
overview 159–61
premenstrual syndrome 160–1
urethral syndrome 162

Hahnemann, Dr Samuel 68
Hamamelis 127
hands-on therapies *see* massage; osteopathy;
    reflexology; Reiki healing
Hatha yoga 111, 112
hay fever 47, 148–9
headaches
    anxiety 7, 8
    herbal medicine 65
    homeopathy 73, 74, 75
    massage 83, 84, 85
    meditation 88
    nutritional medicine 117
    osteopathy and chiropractic 93, 94, 95
    overview 155–7
    Reiki healing 106
    sinusitis 151
    stress 15
health and lifestyle *see* lifestyle management
heart problems
    cardiology 134
    CHD 88, 89, 98, 118, 137
    death and dying 28, 35
    depression 21
    lifestyle management 117, 118
    massage 86
    palliative care 175
    prayer 98
    stress 17
    traditional Chinese medicine 110
Hepar sulphuris 140, 142, 151
hepatitis 74, 142, 175
herbal medicine
    anxiety 8
    aromatherapy 49, 50
    asthma 135
    Ayurvedic medicine 53, 54
    backache 129
    benign prostatic hypertrophy 136
    depression 23
    dermatology 140, 142, 143, 144
    ear, nose and throat 148, 150, 152, 153
    evidence 64–5, 190, 191
    haemorrhoids 127
    inflammatory bowel disease 127
    irritable bowel syndrome 126
    leg cramps 130
    myalgic encephalomyelitis 130
    obstetrics and gynaecology 158, 159, 161, 164
    osteoarthritis and rheumatoid arthritis 128
    overview 61–7
    paediatric medicine 168
    traditional Chinese medicine 108, 109, 110
Heroditus 84
Heron, Barbara 181
Hinduism 31, 112

Hippocrates 2, 50, 61, 68, 137, 192
Hippocratic oath 28
Hittleman, Richard 111
HIV (human immunodeficiency virus) 175
holistic approach
    anxiety 7
    aromatherapy 49
    asthma 134
    Ayurvedic medicine 53
    chronic disease management 125, 126
    death and dying 28
    depression 22
    evidence-based medicine 181, 182, 185, 190,
        199
    homeopathy 68, 69
    integrated health care 1
    massage 84
    spiritual health 121
    yoga 111
Holland, Henry Scott 41
homeopathy 68–77
    anxiety 8, 9, 11, 12
    asthma 135, 170
    backache 129
    benign prostatic hypertrophy 136
    bereavement 38
    cardiology 134
    chronic disease 71
    constitutional remedies 71
    contacts 77
    death and dying 34
    depression 23, 25
    dermatology 139, 140–2, 144
    diabetes mellitus 133
    ear, nose and throat 146–9, 150–3, 169
    essential hypertension 136
    evaluation and evidence-based medicine 181,
        182, 190, 191, 192, 194
    haemorrhoids 127
    headaches 156, 157
    herbal medicine 61, 63
    homeopathic remedies 68–9
    homeopathic remedy guide 71–6
    homeopathic treatment 69–71
    inflammatory bowel disease 127
    integrated health care 2
    irritable bowel syndrome 126
    leg cramps 130
    multiple sclerosis 131, 132
    myalgic encephalomyelitis 130
    neuralgias 131
    obstetrics and gynaecology 158–62, 164, 165
    osteoarthritis and rheumatoid arthritis 127,
        128
    osteoporosis 129
    paediatric medicine 167, 168, 169, 170, 173
    pain 70
    palliative care 175–6
    scarlet fever 69–70
    stress 18, 19
    symptom complex 71
    thyroid disorders 132–3
hormone replacement therapy (HRT) 135, 163,
    164
hormones 22, 45, 49, 101

hospices
    aromatherapy 49
    counselling 57
    death and dying 28, 29, 31, 33, 35, 36, 38
    massage 84
    palliative care 174, 178
hospitals
    aromatherapy 49
    counselling 57
    death and dying 28, 29, 31, 32, 36
    massage 84
    osteopathy 95
    palliative care 174
hot flushes
    homeopathy 70, 73, 75, 175
    menopause 163, 164, 165
    osteoarthritis and rheumatoid arthritis 128
    palliative care 175
housing 115
HRT *see* hormone replacement therapy
humour 19, 24
Huntley Mount Medical Centre (HMMC),
        Bury 181, 185, 194, 198, 199
hyperactivity 95, 117
Hypericum perforatum *see* St John's wort
hypertension
    anxiety 9
    coronary heart disease 137
    essential hypertension 135–6
    exercise 118
    homeopathy 73
    meditation 88
    reflexology 102
    stress 15, 19
hyperventilation 10, 11
hypnotherapy
    evidence-based medicine 80–1, 181, 182, 194
    hay fever 148
    irritable bowel syndrome 126
    overview 78–82
    paediatric medicine 171
    palliative care 176
    viral warts 141
hypothyroidism 22, 132, 133

IBS *see* irritable bowel syndrome
Ignatia (St Ignatius bean) 8, 11, 23, 38, 73
immune system
    acupuncture 45, 46
    Ayurvedic medicine 54
    eczema 143
    herbal medicine 62, 65
    homeopathy 69, 70
    lifestyle management 116, 117
    osteopathy 95
    palliative care 176
    prayer 98
    premenstrual syndrome 161
    research studies 192
    stress 16, 17
    traditional Chinese medicine 109
immunisation 16, 75, 173
in vitro studies 192
infections
    Ayurvedic medicine 54

herbal medicine 64
nutritional medicine 117
obsessive–compulsive behaviour 12
paediatric medicine 95, 169
palliative care 175
stress 16
infertility 116, 159
inflammatory bowel disease 116, 117, 126–7
influenza 65, 72, 152–3
Ingham, Eunice 101
insomnia
    antenatal care 159
    anxiety 7
    lifestyle management 116, 118
    massage 85, 86
    meditation 88
    Reiki healing 106
    stress 18
    yoga 113
insurance 182
integrated health care
    chronic disease management 125
    context vi, 1–3
    evaluation 184–6
    evidence for complementary therapies 187–
        93
    in general practice 194–9
    palliative care 174–7
    setting up an integrated health service 181–3
interpreters 32
intervention trials 191
Ipecacuanha root (Ipecac) 73, 135, 159, 170
Ireland 30, 40–1
irritable bowel syndrome (IBS)
    anxiety 7
    chronic disease 126
    herbal medicine 62
    homeopathy 74
    hypnotherapy 79, 80
    massage 84, 86
    meditation 88
    nutritional medicine 116
    premenstrual syndrome 160
    Reiki healing 106
    stress 15, 18
    traditional Chinese medicine 109
    yoga 113
Iscador (Mistletoe) 176
Islam 30–1, 39, 87, 120

Jehovah's Witnesses 30
Jenny, Dr Hans 121
joints
    backache 129
    depression 26
    exercise 119
    homeopathy 70
    hypnotherapy 80
    massage 85
    osteoarthritis and rheumatoid arthritis 127
    osteopathy and chiropractic 91, 92, 94
Judaism 30, 39, 87
Judith, Anodea 89, 100, 121
Jung, CG 26, 167
juniper 134, 140, 142

Kabat-Zinn, John 56
Kali arsenicosum 143
Kali bichromium 149, 150
Kali bromatum 140
Kali carbonicum 135, 170
Kali muriaticum 141, 169
Kali phosphoricum 131
Kalmia 131
Keleman, Stanley 83, 86
kelp 140
Khan, Hazrat Inayat 108, 199
King's Fund 189
Kipling, Rudyard 59

Lachesis (Bushmaster snake) 71, 73, 156, 161,
     164
language 32
laryngitis 74, 169
laughter therapy 24
lavender
     aromatherapy 50
     dermatology 140, 142, 144
     ear, nose and throat 149, 150
     essential hypertension 135
     herbal medicine 61
     menopause 165
     myalgic encephalomyelitis 130
learning difficulties 95, 117, 120
leg cramps 130
leg ulcers 144
lemon 130, 149, 150
Leopard's bane see Arnica montana
life expectancy 98
lifestyle management 115–22
     anxiety 8, 9, 12
     chronic disease management 71, 125
     contacts 122
     coronary heart disease 137
     depression 21, 23, 24
     evaluation and evidence-based medicine 186,
          190, 191
     exercise 118–19
     homeopathy 71
     music 120–1
     nutritional medicine 116–18
     overview 115–16
     paediatric medicine 171–2
     relaxation 119–20
     spiritual health 121
     stress 18, 20
'like with like' principle 68, 71, 72
Lillium tigrinum 160
Ling, Henriks 84
Liverpool Care Pathway for the Dying 29
Lowen, Alexander 91
Lycopodium (Club moss)
     anxiety 8, 11
     depression 24
     headaches 156
     homeopathic treatment 71, 74
     sinusitis 151
     stress 18

Macmillan Cancer Support 33, 178
macular degeneration 65, 133

magnesium phosphate (Mag phos) 18, 26, 74,
     129, 131–2, 160, 165
Mandela, Nelson 87
manic depression 21, 23, 27, 105
mantras 88, 97, 112
manuka honey 144
Mao Tse-Tung, Chairman 2
marjoram 130
Maslow, Abraham 56, 57
massage
     aromatherapy 49, 50
     asthma 135
     Ayurvedic medicine 53
     bereavement 38
     catarrh 149
     cerebrovascular accident 130
     death and dying 34
     evidence-based medicine 84–5, 181, 190,
          191, 194
     headaches 156, 157
     leg cramps 130
     obstetrics and gynaecology 158, 161, 164
     osteopathy and chiropractic 93
     overview 83–6
     paediatric medicine 171
     palliative care 177
     reflexology 100–3
     traditional Chinese medicine 108, 109
Materia Medica 69, 71
McCullough, Dr M 98
McTimoney, John 94
ME see myalgic encephalomyelitis
Measure Yourself Medical Outcome Profile
     (MYMOP) 182, 184–5
Medical Act (1858) 182
Medicines and Healthcare products Regulatory
     Agency (MHRA) 67, 69
meditation
     anxiety 8, 11, 13
     Ayurvedic medicine 53, 54
     bereavement 39
     death and dying 31, 34
     essential hypertension 136
     hypnotherapy 78, 79
     lifestyle management 119, 120, 121, 172
     obstetrics and gynaecology 158, 160, 161, 164
     overview 87–90
     paediatric medicine 171, 172
     prayer 97
     stress 18
     traditional Chinese medicine 108
     yoga 111, 112, 113
melatonin 65
memory impairment 16, 22, 23, 26, 65
MEND (Mind, Exercise, Nutrition, Diet) 172
meningitis 92, 155
menopause
     depression 22
     essential hypertension 136
     headaches 156
     herbal medicine 62, 64
     homeopathy 73, 74, 75
     massage 85
     nutritional medicine 117
     obstetrics and gynaecology 163–5

osteoarthritis and rheumatoid arthritis 128
reflexology 102
Reiki healing 106
traditional Chinese medicine 109
yoga 113
menorrhagia 160, 165
Mercurius 144, 151, 169
meridians 45, 46, 47, 84, 126
Mesmer, Franz Anton 78
MHRA *see* Medicines and Healthcare products
    Regulatory Agency
migraines
evidence-based medicine 188
headaches 155, 156
herbal medicine 63, 65
homeopathy 73
nutritional medicine 117
osteopathy and chiropractic 92, 93, 95
premenstrual syndrome 160
reflexology 102
stress 15
Miller, Alice 36
Mind (mental health charity) 14
Mistletoe (Iscador) 176
mobility problems 9, 26, 92, 132
Molière 19
Monkshood *see* Aconite napellis
Moore, Thomas 155
Morbilium 169
morning sickness 117, 159
mourning *see* grief
multiple sclerosis (MS) 131–2
musculoskeletal conditions
anxiety 10
aromatherapy 49, 51
evidence-based medicine 188
exercise 119
massage 83, 85
multiple sclerosis 131, 132
osteopathy and chiropractic 91, 92, 93, 94, 95
reflexology 102
Reiki healing 106
relaxation technique 119–20
music 115, 119, 120–1, 122
Muslims 30–1, 39, 87, 120
myalgic encephalomyelitis (ME) 130
MYMOP *see* Measure Yourself Medical Outcome
    Profile
myrrh 49, 50, 55, 127

nasal polyps 150
National Centre for Complementary and
    Alternative Medicine (NCCAM) 189, 193
National Health Service *see* NHS
National Institute for Health and Clinical
    Excellence (NICE) 187, 188
Natrum carbonicum 141, 169
Natrum muriaticum (sea salt)
asthma 135
bereavement 38
death and dying 34
depression 23, 25
diabetes mellitus 133
ear, nose and throat 146, 150, 151, 152
headaches 156

herbal medicine 63
homeopathic treatment 71, 74
multiple sclerosis 131
Natrum muriaticum (sea salt) 132
palliative care 176
premenstrual syndrome 161
urticaria 139
Natrum sulphuricum 127, 170
Natural Death Centre 35
nausea 10, 73, 81, 84, 159, 175–7
NCCAM *see* National Centre for Complementary
    and Alternative Medicine
neck pain 92, 93, 102, 129, 156, 157
nervous breakdown 17, 37
nervous system 87, 91, 119
neuralgias 73–4, 84–5, 131, 156–7
neurotransmitters 24
NHS (National Health Service)
acupuncture 45
chronic disease management 125
counselling 57
death and dying 29
evidence-based medicine 182, 187–9, 199
integrated health care vi, 2, 3
reflexology 102
NICE *see* National Institute for Health and Clinical
    Excellence
nicotine 80, 116
Nietzsche, Friedrich 173
Nin, Anaïs 102
Nitric acid 127, 141, 169
noradrenaline 15, 24
nursing homes 28, 36
nutmeg 55
nutritional medicine
allergies 139
anxiety 8–9, 11, 12, 13
Ayurvedic medicine 53, 54
bereavement 39
contacts 122, 165
coronary heart disease 137
death and dying 30, 31
depression 23, 26
dermatology 139, 140, 142
diabetes mellitus 133
essential hypertension 135
evidence-based medicine 190, 191
irritable bowel syndrome 126
lifestyle management 115, 116–18, 122,
    171–2
macular degeneration 133
multiple sclerosis 132
obstetrics and gynaecology 159, 160, 165
osteoporosis 129
paediatric medicine 171–2, 173
stress 18, 20
traditional Chinese medicine 108
Nux vomica (Poison nut)
antenatal care 158, 159
bereavement 38
depression 24
ear, nose and throat 148, 151
haemorrhoids 127
headaches 156
homeopathic treatment 71, 74

leg cramps 130
    paediatric medicine 169, 170
    stress 18, 19

O'Donohue, John 28, 45, 118
O'Leary, Daniel 165
obesity 118, 137, 172
observational studies 191
obsessions 7, 11–13, 49
obstetrics and gynaecology 158–66
    antenatal care 158–9
    contacts 166
    cystitis 162
    gynaecology 159–61
    menopause 163–5
    urethral syndrome 162
oestrogen 135, 165
Office of Cancer Complementary and Alternative
        Medicine (OCCAM) 189, 193
omega 3 9, 18, 26, 117, 165
Osho 174
osteoarthritis 127–8, 190
osteopathy 91–6
    Alexander technique 93
    applications 93
    back pain 95–6, 129
    Bowen technique 93
    children 95, 168
    chiropractic 93–4
    contacts 96, 166
    cranial osteopathy 94
    evidence-based medicine 92–3, 190
    headaches 157
    history and evidence 91–2
    overview 91
osteoporosis 117, 129, 164, 165
otitis media 73, 75, 146, 148, 167, 169
Outcome of Depression International Network
        (ODIN) 21

paediatric medicine 167–73
    asthma 170
    behavioural problems 170
    childhood infections 169
    complementary therapies 167
    healthy eating and lifestyle 171–2
    homeopathy and immunisation 173
    infantile colic 168
    pain management 171
    teething 168
    threadworms 168
pain
    acupuncture 45, 46, 47, 175
    antenatal care 158, 159
    anxiety 9
    aromatherapy 49, 50, 51
    death and dying 28, 29, 31, 34
    depression 24, 26
    evidence-based medicine 188
    homeopathy 70, 73, 74
    hypnotherapy 79, 80, 176
    massage 83, 84, 85, 86
    meditation 88, 89
    osteoarthritis and rheumatoid arthritis 128
    osteopathy and chiropractic 91, 92, 93, 94, 95

paediatric medicine 95, 171
    palliative care 174, 175, 176, 177
    prayer 98
    reflexology 101, 102
    Reiki healing 105, 106
    yoga 113
palliative care 174–8
    acupuncture 45, 47
    aromatherapy 49, 50, 51
    complementary therapies 174–7
    contacts 178
    death and dying 28, 29, 35
    evidence-based medicine 188
    massage 84, 85
    meditation 88, 89
    reflexology 102
    Reiki healing 106
    yoga 113
Palmer School of Chiropractic 94
Palmer, Daniel 93–4
palpitations 10, 16, 132, 134, 163
panic attacks 8–11, 13, 15, 58, 88
Paracelsus 104
Pasque flower see Pulsatilla
Passiflora 11
Pasteur, Louis 125
PBC see practice-based commissioning
Pell, Cardinal George 97
Pentecostalists 30
peppermint 126, 127, 134, 147, 150, 152, 159
perfectionism 7, 9, 12, 18, 19, 58, 59
personality type 2, 18, 21, 71–2, 101, 108
Petroleum 142, 143, 148
pets 36, 39
phobias 7, 10, 14, 15, 58, 81
Phosphoric acid 133, 169
Phosphorus 71, 74, 150, 170
physical disease 123–78
    chronic disease 125–38
    dermatology 139–45
    ear, nose and throat 146–54
    headaches 155–7
    obstetrics and gynaecology 158–66
    paediatric medicine 167–73
    palliative care 174–8
physiotherapy 45, 84, 102, 130, 157
Phytolacca 153, 169
pilocarpine 169, 175
pine 150
pinworms 168
placebo 46, 62, 75, 101, 189–91
Plato 84
Pliny 84
Plutarch 146
PMS see premenstrual syndrome
Poison ivy see Rhus toxicodendron
Poison nut see Nux vomica
polyps 75, 150, 160
Pomeranz, Dr Bruce 46
postnatal depression 22, 23, 27, 84, 86
post-viral syndrome see myalgic
        encephalomyelitis
poverty 115, 118
practice-based commissioning (PBC) 2, 182, 189
prayer 30, 31, 34, 39–41, 97–9, 120

pregnancy
  antenatal care 158, 159
  Ayurvedic medicine 55
  herbal medicine 65
  homeopathy 69, 73
  massage 85
  nutritional medicine 116, 118
  osteopathy 95
  traditional Chinese medicine 110
premenstrual syndrome (PMS)
  acne 140–1
  depression 22
  headaches 156
  herbal medicine 64
  homeopathy 73, 74, 75
  massage 85
  nutritional medicine 117
  obstetrics and gynaecology 159, 160–1
  reflexology 102
  Reiki healing 106
  traditional Chinese medicine 109
  yoga 113
prescriptions 197–9
primary care
  acupuncture 45
  anxiety 7
  aromatherapy 49
  chronic disease management 125, 126
  counselling 57, 59
  evidence-based medicine 184–9
  stress 15
The Prince's Foundation for Integrated
      Health 182–3, 189, 193
Protestants 30
psoriasis 73, 116, 143–4
Psorinum 150
psychological illness 5–42
  anxiety 7–14
  bereavement 36–42
  death and dying 28–35
  depression 21–7
  integrated health care 3
  obsessive–compulsive behaviour
      11–13
  panic attacks 10–11
  stress 15–20
psychotherapy 8, 12, 14, 21, 23, 59, 80
Pulsatilla (Pasque flower)
  acne 140
  asthma 135, 170
  ear, nose and throat 148, 149, 150, 151,
      169
  haemorrhoids 127
  headaches 156
  homeopathic treatment 71, 74–5
  obstetrics and gynaecology 158, 159, 160,
      161, 165
  paediatric medicine 169, 170
pyridoxine (vitamin B6) 22, 117, 160
Pyrogenium 152

qi (life energy) 45, 104, 108
quality assurance 189
quality of life 26, 174, 176
Quality Outcomes Framework (QOF) 125

radiotherapy 176
randomised controlled trials 92
reactive depression 21
red clover 140, 143
reflexology
  asthma 135
  backache 129
  death and dying 34
  ear, nose and throat 149, 150
  evidence-based medicine 101–2, 181, 190,
      194
  overview 100–3
  palliative care 177
regression 80
Reiki healing
  anxiety 9–10, 11, 13
  bereavement 39
  depression 23, 25
  evidence-based medicine 181, 190, 194
  headaches 156, 157
  multiple sclerosis 131, 132
  obstetrics and gynaecology 158, 160, 161
  overview 104–7
  palliative care 177
  stress 19
Relate 14, 57, 59
relaxation
  acupuncture 46
  anxiety 8, 9, 10–11, 12, 13
  Ayurvedic medicine 53, 54
  bereavement 38, 39
  death and dying 34
  depression 23, 26
  epilepsy 136
  herbal medicine 62
  hypnotherapy 79, 80, 176
  lifestyle management 9, 115, 116, 119–20,
      121, 172
  massage 85
  meditation 87, 88, 89
  myalgic encephalomyelitis 130
  obstetrics and gynaecology 158, 159, 164
  paediatric medicine 171, 172
  palliative care 176, 177
  reflexology 100, 101
  Reiki healing 105
  stress 15, 16, 17, 18, 19
  traditional Chinese medicine 108
religion
  bereavement 36, 39
  death and dying 29–32
  music 120, 121
  prayer 97–9
  spiritual health 121
repertoirising 69, 72
Replens 165
repressed memories 22, 80
research 2, 189–92 see also evidence-based
      medicine
rheumatism 26, 51, 102
rheumatoid arthritis 85, 127–8
rhinorrhoea 73, 149
Rhododendron 127
Rhus toxicodendron (Poison ivy)
  backache 129

dermatology 139, 142
ear, nose and throat 148, 152
headaches 157
homeopathic treatment 70
osteoarthritis and rheumatoid arthritis 127, 128
paediatric medicine 169
ringworm 51
Rinpoche, Sogyal 87
Rogers, Carl 56, 57
Roman, Sanaya 65
rose 50, 165
rose hip syrup 50
rose of opium 50
rosemary 61, 134
Royal College of General Practitioners 29
Royal College of Physicians 29
rubric 72
Ruta 9, 70, 129

Sabadilla 149
Sabal serulata 136
SAD *see* seasonal affect disorder
sage 164, 165
Sai Baba 105
St Ignatius bean *see* Ignatia
St John's wort (Hypericum perforatum)
depression 23
herbal medicine 62, 65
homeopathy 70, 73
multiple sclerosis 131
myalgic encephalomyelitis 130
obstetrics and gynaecology 158, 164
The Samaritans 27, 42
Sambucas 170
sandalwood 142, 144
SANDS (Stillbirth and Neonatal Death Society) 42
Sanguinaria 149, 150
Sarsaparilla 162
Saw palmetto 65, 136
scarlet fever 69, 70, 167
sciatica 70, 73, 74, 93, 129
screening 125, 126, 186
sea salt *see* Natrum muriaticum
seasonal affect disorder (SAD) 25, 27, 65
self-esteem 12, 15, 16
self-help 2, 8, 39, 87
self-hypnosis 79, 80
Seligman, Professor Martin 97
Sepia (Cuttlefish ink)
depression 23, 25
dermatology 140, 141
headaches 156
homeopathic treatment 71, 75
obstetrics and gynaecology 159, 160, 161, 164
osteoarthritis and rheumatoid arthritis 128
serotonin 24, 65
Seventh Day Adventists 30
Shiatsu massage 84, 181, 194
Shine, Betty 37
shock 22, 32, 37, 38, 72, 83
Sikhism 31
Silica 12, 158, 168
Silicea 133, 140, 151

silver nitrate *see* Argentum nitricum
single regeneration budget (SRB) 181, 194
single-blind studies 191
sinuses 51, 75, 95, 100, 102, 150–1, 157
skin conditions 51, 85, 134, 139–45
sleep
anxiety 7, 8, 9, 11, 12, 13
death and dying 34, 38, 39
depression 24, 26
homeopathy 74
hypnotherapy 79
lifestyle management 9, 116, 118, 119
menopause 164
osteopathy 95
palliative care 177
reflexology 101
Reiki healing 105
stress 18, 19
Slippery elm 127
Smallwood report 187, 188
smoking 20, 54, 80, 115–16, 133, 137, 199
Socrates 57, 84
sound 120–1
Spanish fly *see* Cantharis
Spigelia 131
spinal problems 91–4, 129, 175
spirituality
bereavement 36
death and dying 28, 29, 31
lifestyle management 115, 120, 121
music 120, 121
palliative care 174
prayer 97–9
spiritual health 115, 121, 174
sports 84, 85, 86, 94
SRB *see* single regeneration budget
Staphysagria (Stavesacre) 8, 24–5, 71, 75, 137, 162
steroids 69, 148
Stevenson, Robert Louis 13
Still, Dr Andrew T 91, 92
stillbirth 36, 42
stress 15–20
acupuncture 45
anxiety 9, 10, 11
aromatherapy 49, 51
asthma 134
Ayurvedic medicine 54
causes 16–17
contacts 20
coronary heart disease 137
counselling 58
depression 21, 22, 24
essential hypertension 135
evidence-based medicine 181, 187, 188
headaches 157
homeopathy 74, 175
lifestyle management 117, 119
management 17–19
massage 83, 86
meditation 87, 88
multiple sclerosis 131
negative outcomes 17
obstetrics and gynaecology 159, 160, 161
osteopathy and chiropractic 93, 94

overview 15–16
palliative care 175, 177
positive outcomes 17
prayer 98
reflexology 102
Reiki healing 106
symptoms 16
yoga 113
stroke 21, 85, 137
subdural haematoma 155
succussion 68, 69, 192
suicide 17, 22, 23, 27, 36, 58
Sulphur
    depression 25
    dermatology 139, 140, 142, 143
    essential hypertension 136
    haemorrhoids 127
    homeopathic treatment 71, 75
    obstetrics and gynaecology 160, 164
    osteoarthritis and rheumatoid arthritis 128
    paediatric medicine 169
    stress 18, 19
supplements 9, 26, 109, 117, 132, 165
surgery 79, 98, 105, 115, 175–6, 190–1
Sutherland, Dr William 92, 94
Swedish massage 84
symptom complex 69, 71–5, 176
syphilis 86

Tai Chi 108
Takata, Mrs Hayayo 104
tamoxifen 175, 176
Taoist philosophy 45
Tauler, Johannes 177
TCM see traditional Chinese medicine
tea 8, 62, 117, 152, 165
tea-tree oil 51, 140
teething 73, 167, 168
temporal arteritis 155, 156
tennis elbow 93, 94
TENS see transcutaneous electrical nerve
    stimulation
tension headaches 15, 94, 155, 156
Teresa, Mother 55
terminal illness 28, 29, 36, 84 see also death and
    dying; palliative care
therapies, health and lifestyle 43–122
    acupuncture 45–8
    aromatherapy 49–52
    Ayurvedic medicine 53–5
    counselling 56–60
    health and lifestyle 115–22
    herbal medicine 61–7
    homeopathy 68–77
    hypnotherapy 78–82
    integrated health care 3
    massage 83–6
    meditation 87–90
    osteopathy and chiropractic 91–6
    prayer 97–9
    reflexology 100–3
    Reiki healing 104–7
    traditional Chinese medicine 108–10
    yoga 111–14
threadworms 168

Thuja 12, 71, 75, 141, 150, 169
thyme 135, 149, 150
thyroid disorders 10, 132–3
thyroid function tests (TFTs) 10, 133
TIA see transient ischaemic attack
touch therapies 26, 34, 49–51, 177 see also
    massage; osteopathy; reflexology; Reiki
    healing
traditional Chinese medicine (TCM) 45, 61, 92,
    100, 108–10, 142, 190
training 182, 183
tranquillisers 17, 38
Transcendental Meditation UK 90
transcutaneous electrical nerve stimulation
    (TENS) 101
transient ischaemic attack (TIA) 9, 130
trauma 21, 22, 72, 83, 156, 157
travel sickness 147–8
Trungpa, Chogyam 115
tuberculosis (TB) 86

ulcerative colitis see inflammatory bowel disease
ulcers 17, 74, 144
Upanishads 112
upper respiratory tract infections 151–2, 167,
    169
urethral syndrome 162
urinary infections 73, 137, 162
urine therapy 53
Urtica urens 139
urticaria 47, 74, 139–40
Usio, Dr Mikao 104

vaginitis 165
Valnet, Dr J 50
Vedas 112
vertigo 72, 146–7
Vervain 130, 164
viral warts 141–2
vitamins
    anxiety 9
    depression 22, 26
    lifestyle management 117, 171
    macular degeneration 133
    obstetrics and gynaecology 160, 165
    stress 18
Vitex agnus castus (VAC) 64
vomiting 70, 81, 167, 175, 176

wakes 30, 40–1
warts 75, 141–2, 169
water intake see fluid intake
weight management 22, 25, 95, 113, 118, 135,
    172
wheatgerm 165
Whitman, Walt 28
WHO see World Health Organization
Wild hops see Bryonia
wild oats 130
Wild yam 164
Willow bark 129, 148
wills 33
wintergreen 134
witch hazel 127
work 9, 15, 16, 18, 19, 185–6

World Health Organization (WHO) vi, 62, 189, 193

worms 64, 168

X-ray 93

yang 45, 108, 111
yarrow 140, 152, 153
yin 45, 108, 111
yoga
    anxiety 8, 11, 13
    Ayurvedic medicine 53, 54
    depression 25
    lifestyle management 119, 172
    meditation 87
    obstetrics and gynaecology 158, 164
    osteoporosis 129
    overview 111–14
    stress 18
Yudkin, Professor John 117

zinc 9, 18, 117, 132, 133, 140, 165
Zukav, Gary 21